COLOUR GUIDE

PICTURE TESTS

Imaging

Jeremy Hughes MA PhD MRCP

Lecturer in Medicine, University Hospital,
Nottingham, UK

Michael Hughes FRCS Ed. FRCR

Consultant Radiologist, Warwick Hospital,
Warwick, UK

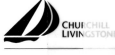

CHURCHILL LIVINGSTONE

NEW YORK, EDINBURGH, LONDON, MADRID, MELBOURNE,
SAN FRANCISCO AND TOKYO

CHURCHILL LIVINGSTONE
Medical Division of Pearson Professional Limited

Distributed in the United States of America by Churchill
Livingstone Inc., 650 Avenue of the Americas, New York,
N.Y. 10011, and by associated companies, branches and
representatives throughout the world.

©Pearson Professional Limited 1997

First published 1997

ISBN 0-443-05591-2

British Library of Cataloguing in Publication Data
A catalogue record for this book is available from the British
Library.

Library of Congress Cataloging in Publication Data
A catalog record for this book is available from the Library
of Congress.

Publisher
Laurence Hunter

Project Editor
Jim Killgore

Production
Nancy Arnott

Design Direction
Erik Bigland

Produced by Longman Asia Limited, Hong Kong
SWT/01

Preface

This book is primarily intended for medical students, although doctors preparing for postgraduate examinations such as the MRCP will find it useful. Hospital practitioners depend upon the radiology department for many investigations that are crucial to the successful management of patients and this book should serve to emphasise the symbiotic relationship which exists between radiology and medicine.

Nottingham   J.H.
Warwick   M.H.
1997

Acknowledgements

This book is dedicated to our parents, wives (Brenda [JH] and Caroline [MH]) and children (Lloyd, Owen and Rhian [JH] and Charlotte, Rebecca and Edward [MH]) for their patience during the preparation of this book. We are very grateful to Professor PC Rubin, Professor JR Hampton and Dr SD Ryder for permission to use their radiographs. MH is very grateful for the encouragement of colleagues and staff at Warwick hospital and would like to thank Alliance Medical for their technical assistance with some of the magnetic resonance images.

Contents

Questions

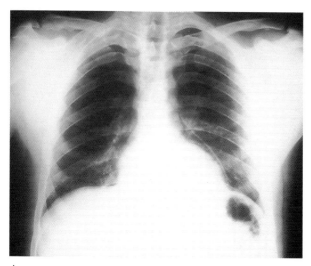

1. **This chest X-ray is of a 48-year-old man who has been involved in a road traffic accident.**

a. Describe the abnormality.
b. What is the diagnosis?

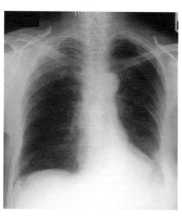

2. **This is a chest X-ray of a 63-year-old woman who previously underwent a right mastectomy for breast carcinoma (no radiotherapy) and who has now developed a right Horner's syndrome.**

a. What is Horner's syndrome?
b. Describe the radiological abnormality.
c. Suggest a diagnosis.

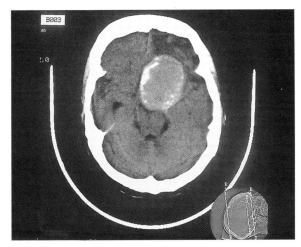

A

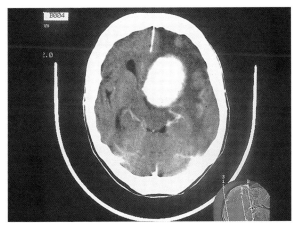

B

3. **(A) and (B) are CT brain scans (pre- and post-intravenous contrast, respectively) of a 48-year-old man who presented with headaches, slurred speech and incontinence.**

a. Describe the abnormalities.
b. Suggest a diagnosis.
c. What treatment is advisable?

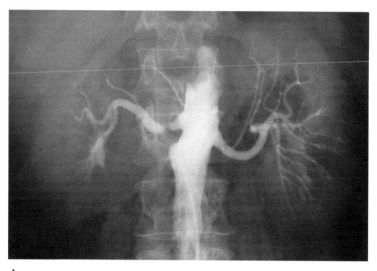

4. a. What is this investigation?
 b. Describe the abnormality.
 c. How may this patient have presented?
 d. What treatment may be offered?

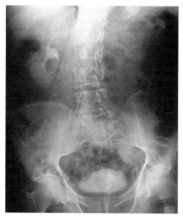

5. This intravenous urogram is from a 68-year-old man who had undergone no previous surgery and who was referred to medical outpatients with persistent dipstick proteinuria and haematuria and normal renal function.

a. Describe the abnormality.
b. What further investigations are indicated?

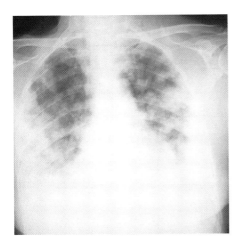

6. This is a chest X-ray of a 66-year-old man who is short of breath.

a. Describe the abnormality.
b. Give a differential diagnosis.
c. What treatment is available?

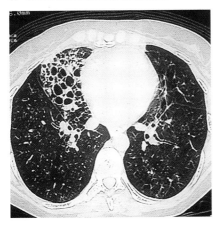

7. This is a high-resolution lung CT scan of a 62-year-old man.

a. Describe the abnormality.
b. What condition does this patient have?
c. Suggest 3 causes.
d. What complications can occur?

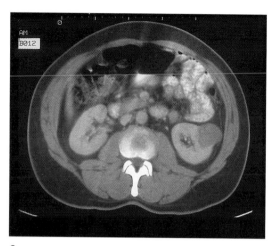

8. This is an abdominal CT scan of a 54-year-old man.

a. Describe the abnormality.
b. What is the diagnosis?
c. How may this condition present?

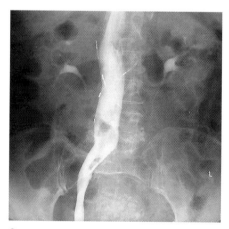

9. This X-ray was performed on a 68-year-old woman.

a. What procedure has been performed?
b. In what circumstances may this be useful?

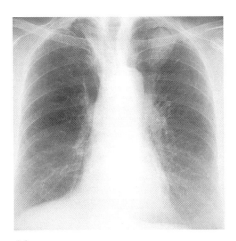

10. This is a chest X-ray of a 79-year-old woman who was referred to the outpatient clinic following an episode of haemoptysis.

a. Describe the abnormality.
b. What is the diagnosis?
c. What further tests may be useful?
d. What treatment is required?

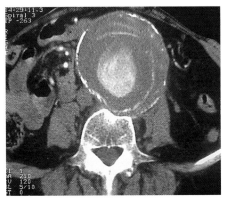

11. This is a contrast-enhanced abdominal CT scan of a 67-year-old man.

a. What is the diagnosis?
b. What symptoms may the patient complain of?
c. Give three predisposing factors.
d. What treatment is available?

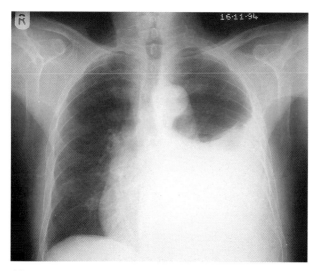

12. This is a chest X-ray of an 83-year-old man who complains of shortness of breath on exertion.

a. What is the main abnormality?
b. Give a differential diagnosis.
c. What further investigations are indicated?

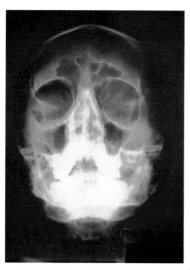

13. This patient was assaulted and had considerable facial swelling.

a. What does the plain film demonstrate?
b. What is its significance?

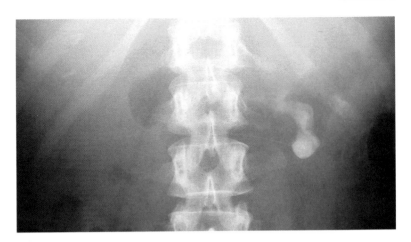

14. This abdominal X-ray is of a 24-year-old woman who has a history of recurrent urinary tract infections.

a. Describe the abnormality and suggest a diagnosis.
b. Is there any association between this condition and urinary tract infections?
c. What treatment may be offered?

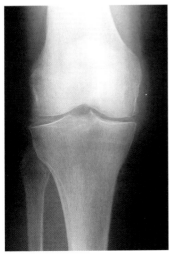

15. This X-ray is of the right knee of a 54-year-old woman who experiences intermittent episodes of acute knee discomfort.

a. Describe the abnormality.
b. What condition does this patient have?
c. Give two associated conditions.
d. Outline the treatment.

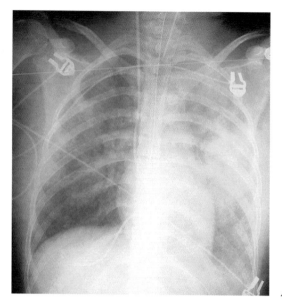

A

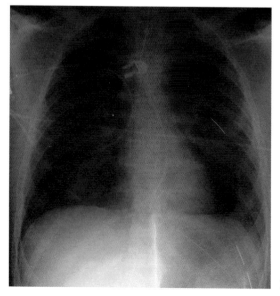

B

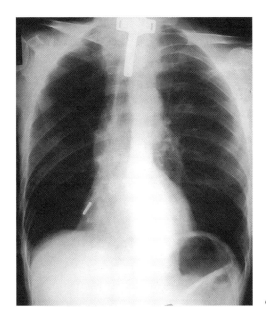

C

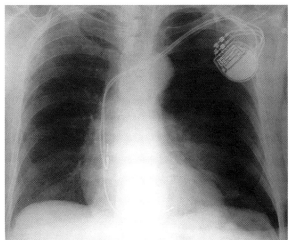

D

16. These routine chest X-rays are from patients who have undergone invasive procedures.

a. Describe the abnormality in each case.

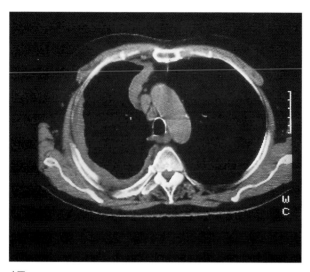

17. This is a thoracic CT scan of a 60-year-old retired shipyard worker.

a. Describe the abnormality.
b. What is the most likely diagnosis?
c. Suggest an underlying cause.
d. What physical signs may be present?
e. What treatment is available?

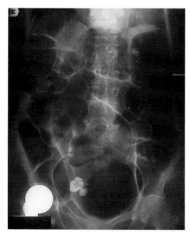

18. This abdominal X-ray is of an 81-year-old woman who was admitted with marked abdominal swelling.

a. Describe the abnormality.
b. What is the radiological diagnosis and why?
c. What treatment may be given?

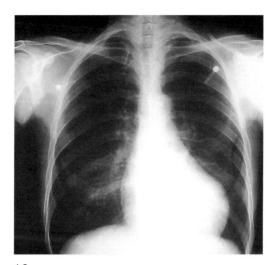

19. This chest X-ray is of a 64-year-old smoker.

a. Describe the main abnormality.
b. What is the diagnosis?
c. How may this man have presented?
d. What treatment may be required?

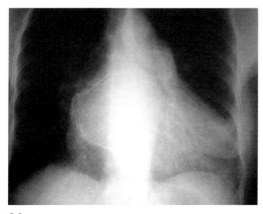

20. This penetrated chest X-ray is of a 69-year-old man.

a. Describe the abnormality and suggest a cause.

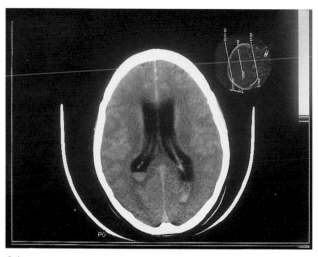

21. This is a CT brain scan of a 44-year-old woman who was found unconscious at home. She was hypoxic on air with widespread bilateral inspiratory crackles.

a. Describe the abnormality.
b. What is the diagnosis and why is she hypoxic?
c. What treatment is available?

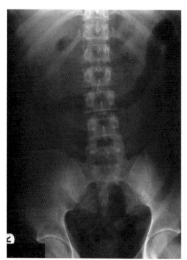

22. This abdominal X-ray is of a 36-year-old man with long-standing diarrhoea.

a. Describe the abnormality.
b. What is the diagnosis?
c. What are the complications of this condition?

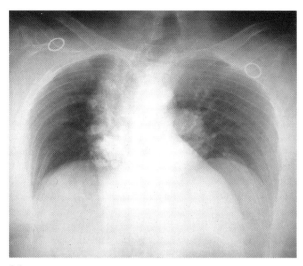

23. This is a chest X-ray of a 68-year-old woman who complains of shortness of breath, morning headaches and ankle oedema.

a. Describe the abnormality.
b. What is the most likely diagnosis?
c. What further investigation is required?
d. What treatment may be given?

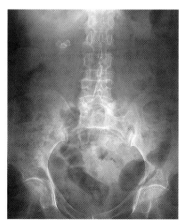

24. This abdominal X-ray is of a 65-year-old woman who has a history of intermittent abdominal pain with vomiting.

a. Describe the abnormality and suggest a diagnosis.
b. What other complications can occur?
c. What treatment may be offered?

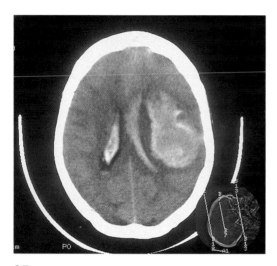

25. This is a CT brain scan of a 69-year-old woman who collapsed while shopping.

a. Describe the abnormalities and give a diagnosis.
b. Give three predisposing conditions.

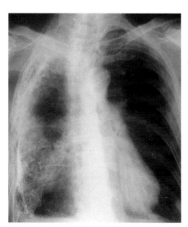

26. This chest X-ray is of a 65-year-old man.

a. Describe the abnormality and suggest a cause.

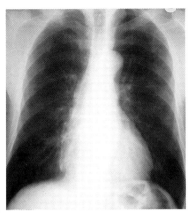
A

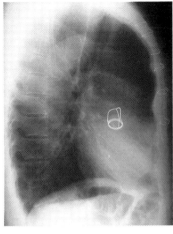
B

27. These chest X-rays are of a 60-year-old man.

a. Describe the abnormality.
b. Give three possible reasons for the surgery.
c. What complications may arise?
d. What was the phase of the cardiac cycle when the X-rays were taken?

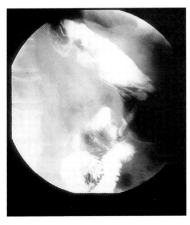

28. This patient has a long history of a gastric ulcer, and was given a barium meal to investigate more recent weight loss and anaemia.

a. What does this single view from the barium meal demonstrate?
b. What is the next investigation?

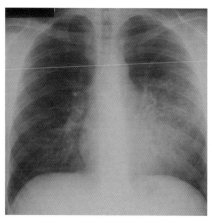
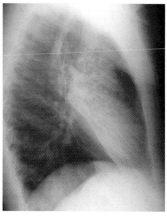

A   B

29. **These chest X-rays are of a febrile 38-year-old pet shop owner.**

a. Describe the abnormality.
b. Give a differential diagnosis.
c. What treatment should he receive?

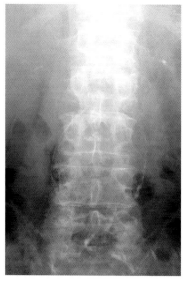

30. **This X-ray of a 72-year-old man with back pain was arranged by his GP.**

a. Describe the abnormality and suggest a cause.
b. What should the GP do?

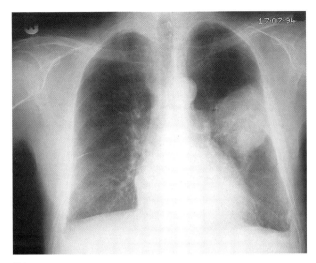

31. This is a chest X-ray of a 61-year-old man undergoing investigations for weight loss.

a. Describe the abnormality.
b. What is the most likely diagnosis?
c. What may blood tests show?
d. What further investigation is required?
e. What treatment may be given?

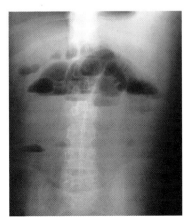

32. This erect abdominal X-ray is of a 54-year-old woman who presented to casualty with abdominal pain and vomiting.

a. Describe the abnormality and suggest a diagnosis.
b. What physical signs may be present?
c. Give three causes.
d. What treatment should be instituted?

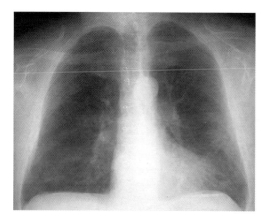

33. This chest X-ray is of a 50-year-old man.

a. Describe the abnormality and suggest a cause.

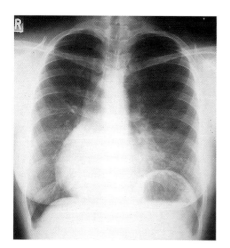

34. This is a pre-employment chest X-ray of a 25-year-old woman.

a. Describe the abnormality.
b. What would the electrocardiograph show?
c. What questions would you ask the patient?

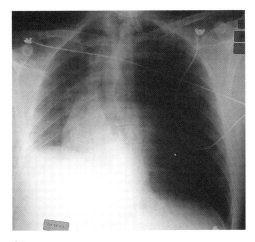

35. This chest X-ray is of a previously fit 24-year-old man.

a. Describe the abnormality and give the diagnosis.
b. Should this X-ray have been performed?

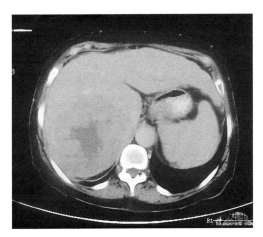

36. This is an abdominal CT scan of a 59-year-old alcoholic.

a. Describe the abnormality.
b. Suggest a diagnosis.
c. Give two predisposing factors.
d. What treatment is available?

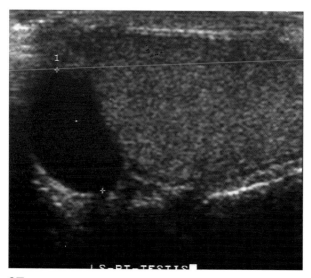

37. This middle-aged man had a painless scrotal swelling on the right side and was referred for further investigation.

a. What does the ultrasound scan show?
b. What would you advise next?

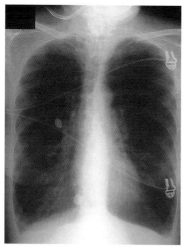

38. This chest X-ray was performed in a 62-year-old woman recovering from a chest infection.

a. Describe the abnormalities.
b. What is the underlying pulmonary condition?
c. What is the usual underlying cause?
d. What physical signs may be present?

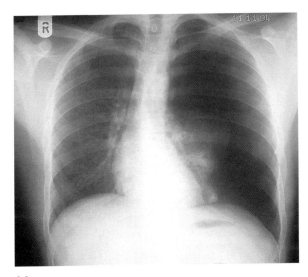

39. This is a chest X-ray of a 20-year-old young man.

a. Describe the abnormality.
b. What is the diagnosis?
c. Suggest three causes.
d. What treatment is required?

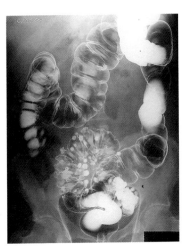

40. This barium enema is from a 65-year-old woman.

a. Describe the obvious abnormality.
b. What complications may occur?
c. Outline the management.

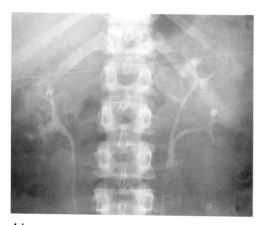

41. This intravenous urogram is from a 56-year-old man who has had two episodes of transient macroscopic haematuria.

a. Describe the abnormality.
b. Does it explain his symptoms?
c. Are any further investigations indicated?

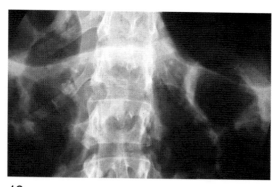

42. This abdominal X-ray is of a 50-year-old man with chronic abdominal pain and weight loss.

a. Describe the abnormality.
b. What is the diagnosis?
c. Suggest three causes.
d. What treatment can be given?

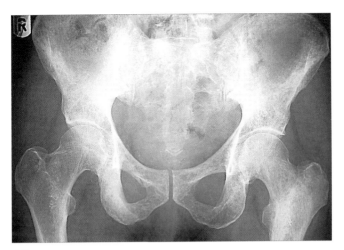

43. This pelvic X-ray is from a 66-year-old man whose buttock was bruised following a fall.

a. Describe the abnormality.
b. What is the differential diagnosis?
c. What blood tests may be abnormal in this patient?

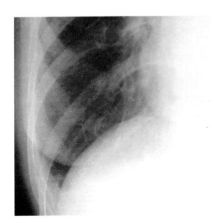

44. This is a close-up view of the right lower zone of a chest X-ray of a 58-year-old woman.

a. Describe the abnormality.
b. Give two causes.

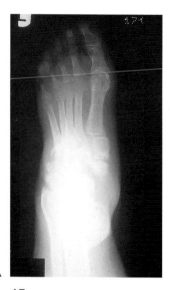
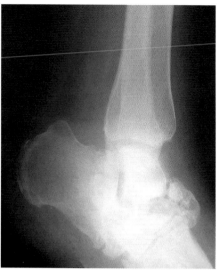

A

B

45. **These X-rays are of the left foot of a 54-year-old man. There is no history of infection.**

a. Describe the abnormality.
b. Suggest a diagnosis.

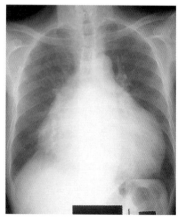

46. This is a chest X-ray of a 61-year-old, alcoholic, non-smoking man who complains of exertional dyspnoea.

a. Describe the abnormality.
b. What physical signs may be present?
c. What treatment is required?

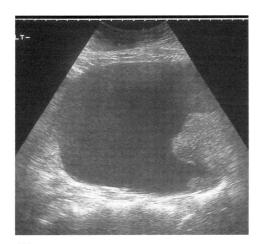

47. This is a pelvic ultrasound of a 53-year-old woman with a palpable pelvic mass.

a. Describe the abnormality and suggest a diagnosis.
b. What treatment is available?

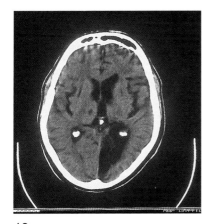

48. This is a CT brain scan of a 65-year-old man who was referred from his GP for assessment of 'dementia'.

a. Describe the abnormalities.
b. Suggest an underlying cause.

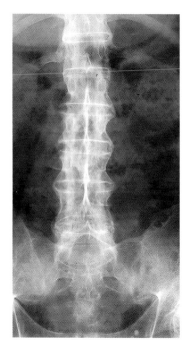

49. This X-ray is of a 54-year-old man with a long history of arthritis.

a. Describe the abnormality.
b. Suggest a diagnosis.
c. Give two associated conditions.

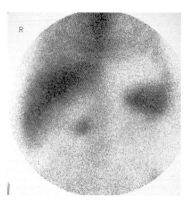

50. This white cell scan (anterior view) is from a 40-year-old man undergoing investigations for a pyrexia of unknown origin.

a. What is demonstrated?
b. Suggest a cause.
c. What treatment is indicated?

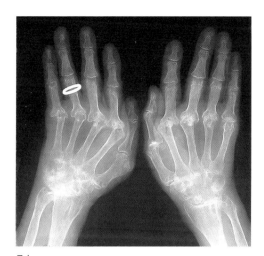

51. **This X-ray of the hands is from a lady with long-standing arthritis.**

a. Describe at least three abnormalities.
b. Suggest two diagnoses that could produce this radiological appearance.
c. What physical signs would help to distinguish between them?

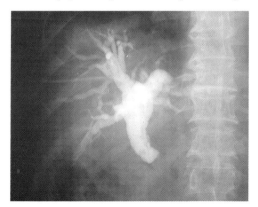

52. **This investigation is from a 62-year-old man.**

a. What procedure has been performed?
b. Describe the abnormality and suggest a diagnosis.
c. How may the patient have presented?

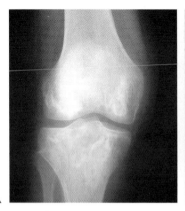 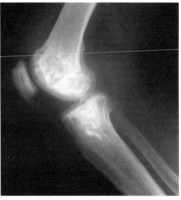

A

B

53. These X-rays are of a 59-year-old woman's knee.

a. Describe the abnormality.
b. What is the diagnosis?
c. Give two predisposing conditions.

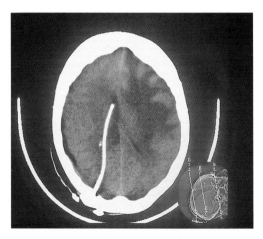

54. This is a CT brain scan of a 56-year-old man with a left glioma (not shown).

a. What procedure has been performed?
b. What are the associated complications of this procedure?

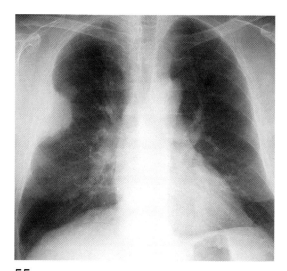

55. This chest X-ray is of a 58-year-old man who has had persistent right-sided chest pain for several weeks.

a. Describe the abnormality.
b. Suggest a diagnosis.

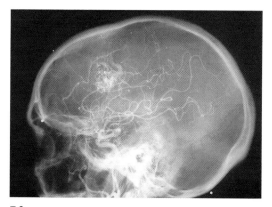

56. This is a left carotid arteriogram of a 36-year-old man.

a. Describe the abnormality.
b. Give two potential complications.

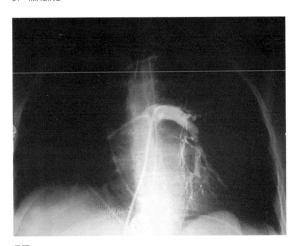

57. a. What is this investigation?
   b. What is the diagnosis?
   c. Give four predisposing causes.

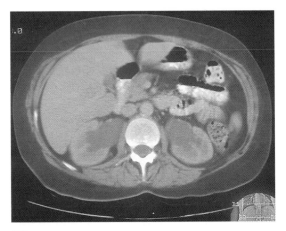

58. **This is an abdominal CT scan of a 50-year-old man.**

a. Describe the abnormality.
b. What symptoms may he have presented with?
c. Suggest three causes.

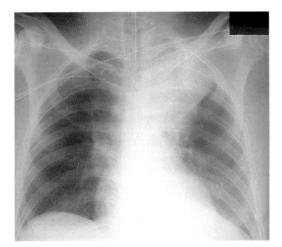

59. This chest X-ray is of a 48-year-old man in the intensive care department. His oxygen saturation has just fallen.

a. Describe the abnormality and suggest a cause.
b. Outline treatment.

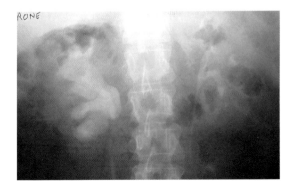

60. This intravenous urogram is from a 26-year-old woman who has intermittent episodes of right-sided loin pain.

a. Describe the abnormality and suggest a diagnosis.
b. What is the aetiology?
c. What treatment can be offered?

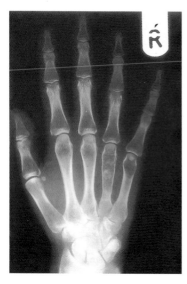

61. **This is a hand radiograph from a young man experiencing minor discomfort in the palm region.**

a. What does this hand radiograph demonstrate?
b. Describe a common presentation.
c. Is this a typical site?

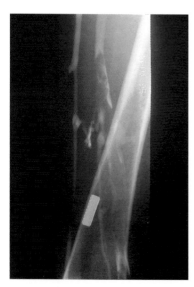

62. **This investigation was performed in a 59-year-old man who had recently been unwell with influenza.**

a. What is this investigation?
b. Describe the abnormality and suggest a diagnosis.
c. What treatment should be given?

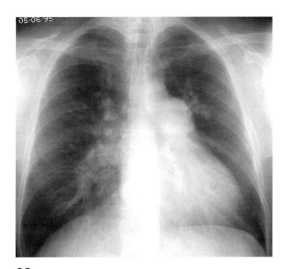

63. This chest X-ray is of a 44-year-old man who has developed atrial fibrillation.

a. Describe the abnormality.
b. What is the most likely diagnosis?
c. What physical signs may be present?
d. What further investigations are required?

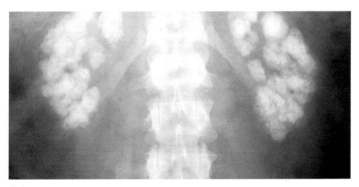

64. This plain abdominal X-ray is of a 38-year-old man who complained of a sudden onset of right-sided abdominal pain. A full biochemical profile was normal.

a. Describe the abnormality and suggest a diagnosis.
b. What is the cause of his abdominal pain?

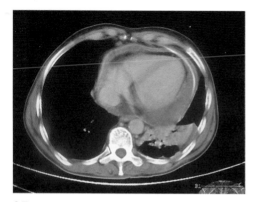

65. This is a chest CT scan of a 55-year-old smoker.

a. Describe the abnormalities.
b. Suggest two possible diagnoses.
c. What treatment has been given?

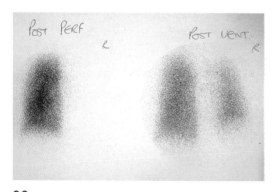

66. This ventilation–perfusion scan was performed in a young woman.

a. What does it show?
b. What is the diagnosis?
c. How may she have presented?
d. What physical signs may be present?

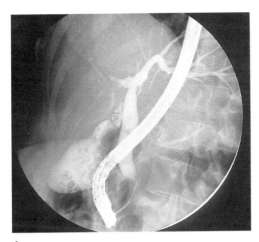

A

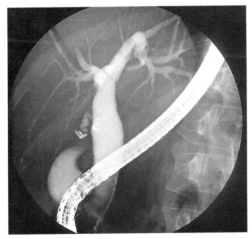

B

67. (A) and (B) are films from endoscopic retrograde cholangiopancreatograms (ERCPs) that were performed 3 years apart on the same patient.

a. Describe the abnormality in (A).
b. What procedure was later performed?

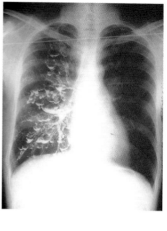

A

B

68. Chest X-ray of a 30-year-old man.

a. Describe the abnormalities in (A).
b. What investigation is shown in (B) and what does it demonstrate?
c. What treatment is available?

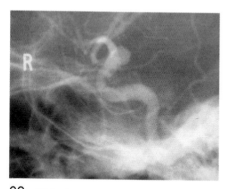

69. This is a cerebral angiogram which has been performed in a 48-year-old woman.

a. Describe the abnormality.
b. Suggest two associated conditions.
c. What treatment may be offered?

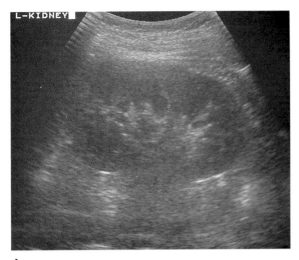

A

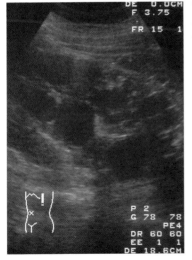

B

70. (A) is a normal renal ultrasound, and (B) is a renal ultrasound examination of a 45-year-old normotensive man.

a. Describe the abnormality in (B).
b. What is the diagnosis?
c. What is the treatment?

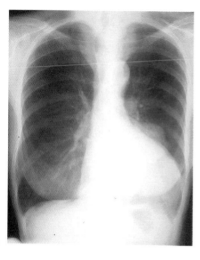
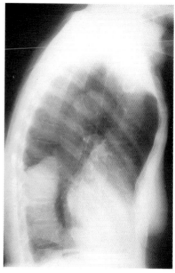

A

B

71. These chest X-rays are of a 66-year-old woman.

a. Describe the abnormality and suggest a cause.

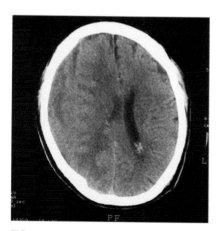

72. This is an image from a 68-year-old man's brain scan. He had a 3-week history of increasing early morning headaches.

a. What does the scan show?
b. What are the possible management options?

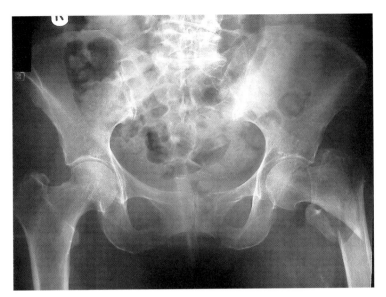

73. This pelvic X-ray is of an 80-year-old woman who is 'off her legs'.

a. Describe the abnormality.
b. What characteristic physical sign is usually present?
c. What treatment is indicated?

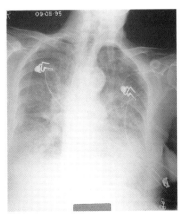

74. This chest X-ray is of an acutely unwell 74-year-old woman.

a. Describe the abnormalities.
b. What is the diagnosis and what treatment may be given?
c. Suggest three possible cardiac causes.

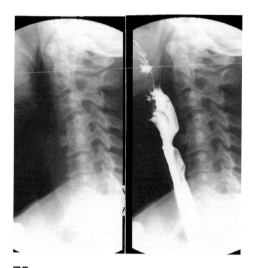

75. This middle-aged lady was having increasing difficulty in swallowing—these symptoms commenced after an orthopaedic neck operation.

a. What operation has been performed?
b. What is the further management?

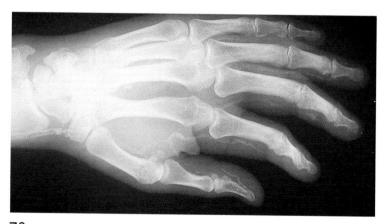

76. This hand X-ray is from a 45-year-old man.

a. Describe the abnormality.
b. What two medical conditions can account for this appearance?

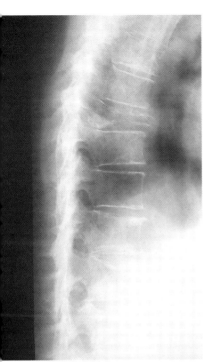

77. This lateral thoracic spine X-ray is of a previously active 71-year-old man who presented with acute back pain. He was found to be hypercalcaemic with mild renal impairment.

a. Describe the abnormality.
b. Suggest a possible diagnosis.
c. What further investigations are indicated?
d. What treatment is available?

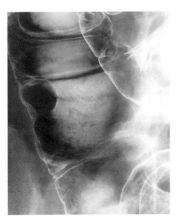

78. This barium enema is from a 39-year-old lady who was referred to outpatients following an episode of mild rectal bleeding.

a. Describe the abnormality and suggest a diagnosis.
b. What treatment is indicated?

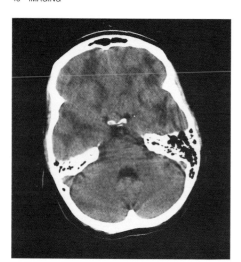

A

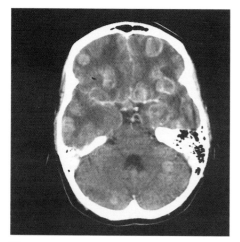

B

79. This 48-year-old lady was initially admitted as an acute psychiatric patient when she was unable to cope at home, becoming increasingly disinhibited in behaviour and disorientated.

a. What does the CT scan demonstrate?
b. What is the likely underlying cause?

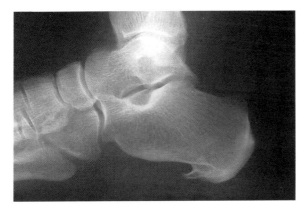

80. This heel X-ray is from a 52-year-old man who complains of pain on walking.

a. What is the diagnosis?
b. What treatment is available?

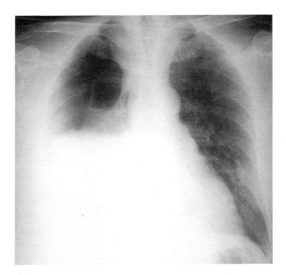

81. This chest X-ray is of a 66-year-old man who complains of shortness of breath and right-sided chest pain.

a. Describe the abnormality.
b. What is the radiological differential diagnosis?
c. What treatment and investigations are indicated?

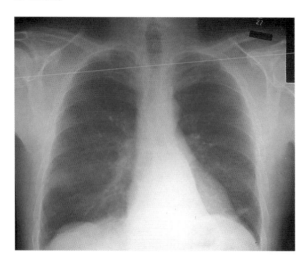

82. This chest X-ray is of a 52-year-old smoker who is slow to recover from a right total hip replacement.

a. Describe the abnormality and give a diagnosis.
b. What physical signs may be present?
c. Suggest a cause.

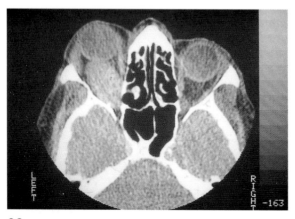

83. This is a CT brain scan of a 67-year-old woman.

a. Describe the abnormality.
b. Give a differential diagnosis.

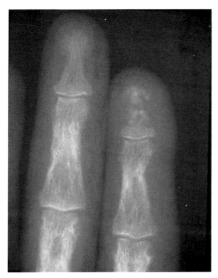
A

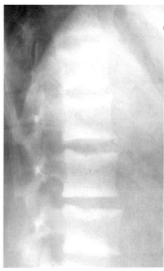
B

84. These X-rays are of a 46-year-old woman who has been on haemodialysis for 18 years.

a. Describe the abnormalities.
b. What is the diagnosis?
c. Outline treatment.

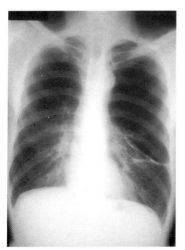

85. This chest X-ray is of a 56-year-old man.

a. Describe the abnormality and give a diagnosis.
b. What physical signs may be present?
c. What treatment is possible?

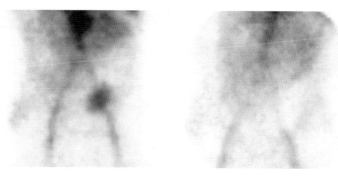

A   B

86. These ⁹⁹ᵐTc-diethylene triamine penta-acetic acid (DTPA) scans were performed in a 39-year-old man 3 days (A) and 9 days (B) following a cadaveric renal transplant.

a. What do they demonstrate?
b. Suggest a cause.
c. What treatment is indicated?

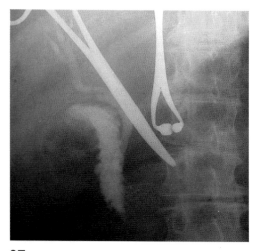

87. This investigation is from a 58-year-old woman.

a. What procedure has been performed and why?

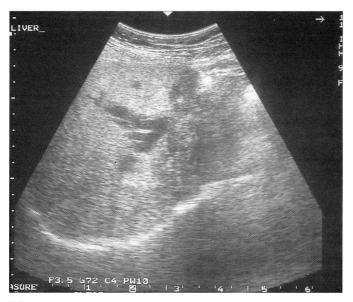

88. This is a liver ultrasound examination of a febrile, icteric 67-year-old woman.

a. Describe the abnormality.
b. Give a differential diagnosis.
c. What further investigations and treatment may be indicated?

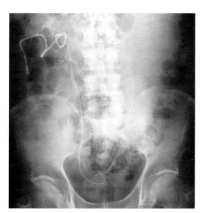

89. This abdominal X-ray is of a 46-year-old diabetic man who presented with right-sided abdominal pain.

a. What procedures have been performed?
b. Suggest a cause.

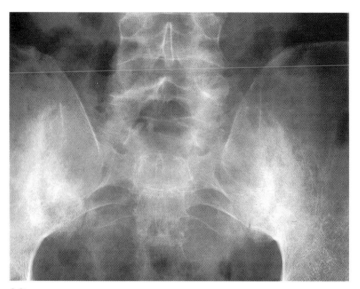

90. This X-ray is of a 42-year-old man with a long history of lower back pain.

a. Describe the abnormality.
b. Give a differential diagnosis.

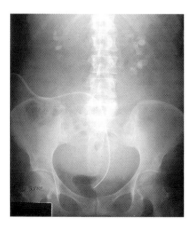

91. This plain abdominal X-ray is of a 66-year-old woman who has had a previous parathyroidectomy.

a. Describe the abnormality and suggest a diagnosis.
b. Give two possible reasons for the parathyroidectomy.

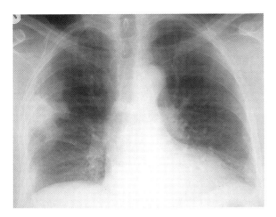

92. This chest X-ray is of an afebrile 48-year-old man who was admitted to hospital with acute chest pain.

a. Describe the abnormality.
b. Suggest a diagnosis.
c. What other investigations would be helpful?

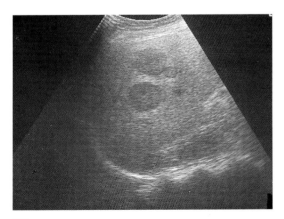

93. This is a liver ultrasound examination of a 65-year-old woman with long-standing ulcerative colitis.

a. Describe the abnormality.
b. Give a differential diagnosis.
c. What further investigations may be indicated?

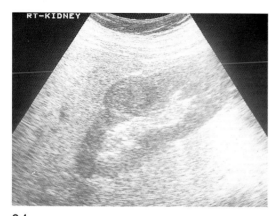

94. This is a renal ultrasound examination of a 55-year-old polycythaemic man.

a. Describe the abnormality.
b. What is the most likely diagnosis?
c. What is the cause of the polycythaemia?
d. What further investigations and treatment may be indicated?

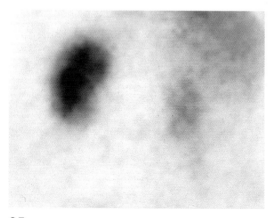

95. This DTPA scan (posterior view) was performed in a 49-year-old woman.

a. What does it demonstrate?
b. Give three causes.

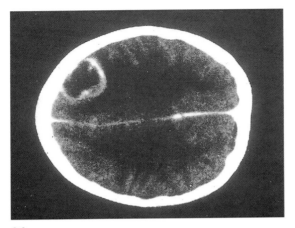

96. This is a contrast-enhanced CT brain scan of a patient with infective endocarditis who suffered an epileptic fit.

a. Describe the abnormality.
b. Suggest a diagnosis.
c. What treatment is indicated?

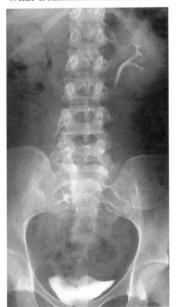

97. This intravenous urogram is of a 40-year-old woman with a serum creatinine of 150 μmol/l and 1.2 g of proteinuria per 24 hours.

a. Describe the abnormality.
b. Does it explain her elevated creatinine and proteinuria?
c. Are any further investigations indicated?

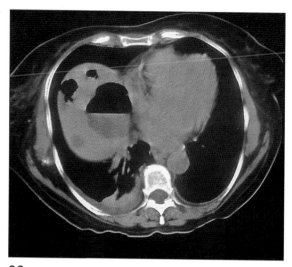

98. This is a lower thoracic/upper abdominal CT scan of a 72-year-old woman who is febrile and toxic.

a. Describe the abnormality.
b. Suggest an underlying cause.
c. What treatment is required?

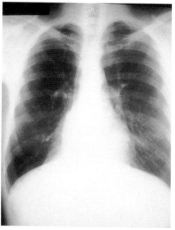

99. This chest X-ray is of a 45-year-old man who developed persistent coughing during and following his evening meal.

a. Describe the abnormality.
b. What further investigation is indicated?

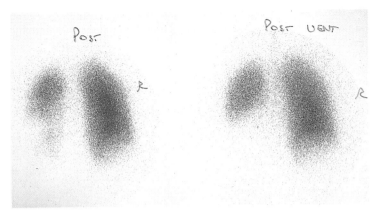

100. This ventilation–perfusion scan was performed in a 28-year-old woman.

a. What does it show?
b. Suggest two causes.

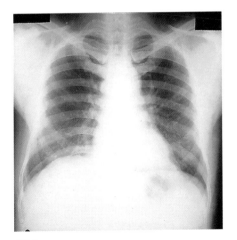

101. This is a pre-operative chest X-ray of an asymptomatic 34-year-old woman.

a Describe the abnormality.
b. What condition has this patient had?
c. Should the anaesthetist be concerned?

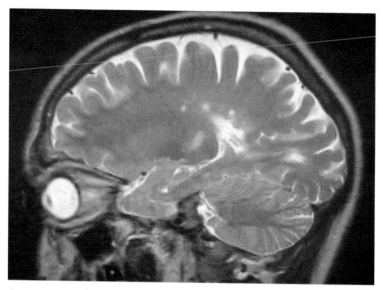

A

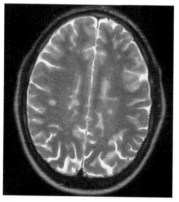

B

102. These MRI scans are from a 35-year-old man with a history of unsteadiness who presented with decreased left visual acuity.

a. Describe the abnormality and suggest a diagnosis.
b. What may be seen on fundoscopy?

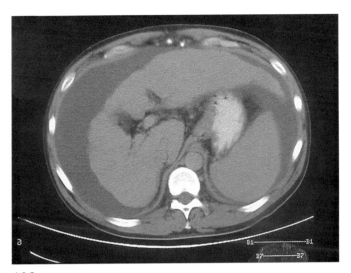

103. This is an abdominal CT scan of a 36-year-old man who presented with abdominal swelling and peripheral oedema.

a. Describe the abnormalities.
b. Suggest a diagnosis.
c. Give three causes.
d. Suggest four useful investigations.

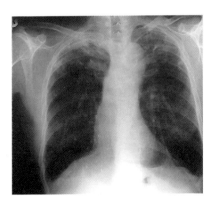

104. This chest X-ray is of a 67-year-old man.

a. Describe the abnormality.
b. What is the diagnosis?

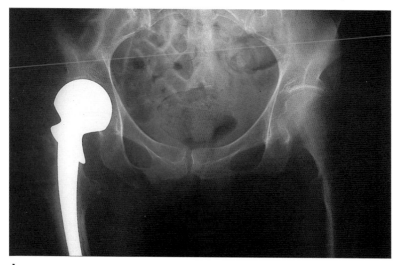

A

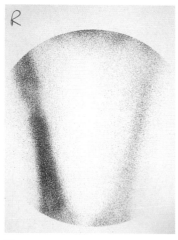

B

105. **(A)** is a plain X-ray and **(B)** is an isotope bone scan, both performed in a 62-year-old woman who was admitted 3 months following a right hemiarthroplasty complaining of night sweats, fever and loss of weight over 2 weeks.

a. What do they demonstrate?
b. Suggest a cause.

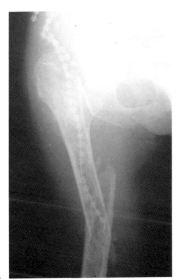 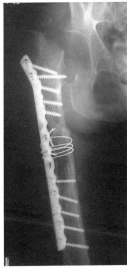

A   B

106. These plain hip X-rays were performed in the same patient as in question 105.

a. What do they demonstrate?

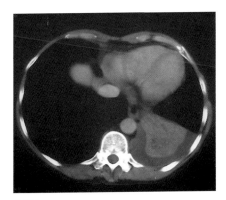

107. This is a chest CT scan of a previously fit 45-year-old non-smoker.

a. Describe the abnormality and suggest a diagnosis.
b. What physical signs may be found in the chest?
c. What further investigations are indicated?

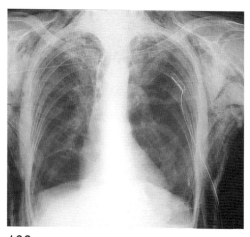

108. This chest X-ray is of a 24-year-old man who has been involved in a road traffic accident.

a. Describe the abnormalities and give the most likely cause.
b. What physical sign will be present?

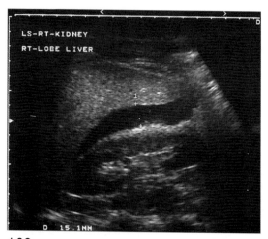

109. This abdominal ultrasound scan was performed in a young man who had been involved in a road traffic accident.

a. What does it demonstrate?
b. What are the possible causes?

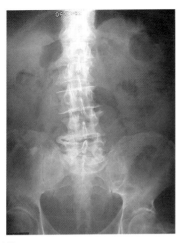
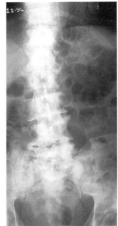

A   B

110. The lumbar spine X-ray on the right is from a man who complains of numerous aches and pains, particularly affecting his back. The X-ray on the left was taken 3 years previously.

a. Describe the abnormality.
b. What further tests are indicated?
c. Outline treatment options.

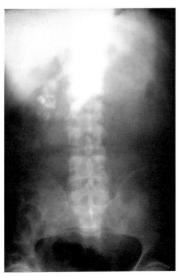

111. This plain abdominal X-ray is of a 36-year-old Asian woman with no history of renal calculi and who has renal impairment.

a. Describe the abnormality and suggest a diagnosis.
b. What other investigations are indicated?

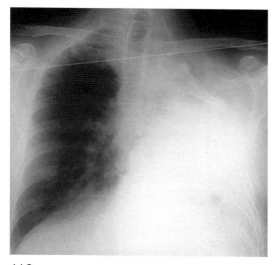

112. This chest X-ray is of a 70-year-old man who is a long-standing attender at the chest clinic.

a. Describe the abnormalities.
b. Suggest a diagnosis.

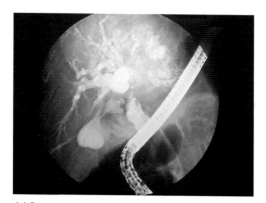

113. This investigation is from a 69-year-old woman.

a. What procedure has been performed?
b. Describe the abnormality.
c. Suggest a differential diagnosis.
d. What can be done to alleviate the patient's symptoms?

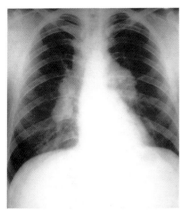

114. This chest X-ray of a 38-year-old man was performed when he started work in the NHS.

a. Describe the abnormality.
b. Give a differential diagnosis.
c. What would pulmonary function tests demonstrate?
d. What further investigations are required?

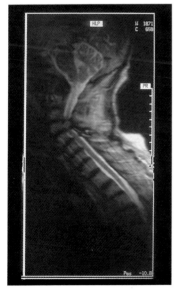

115. This MRI scan is of an 81-year-old man who became increasingly weak and unable to care for himself at home.

a. Describe the abnormality.
b. What physical signs may be present?
c. What treatment is available?

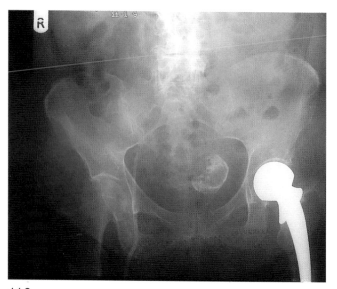

116. This pelvic X-ray is of a 72-year-old woman with acute renal failure.

a. Describe three abnormalities.
b. Are these abnormalities related to each other?

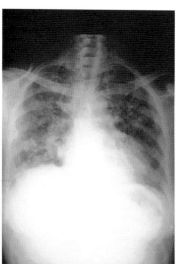

117. This chest X-ray is of a 54-year-old woman with mild persistent hypercalcaemia.

a. Describe the abnormality.
b. Suggest a diagnosis.
c. What other organs may be affected?
d. What treatment is available?

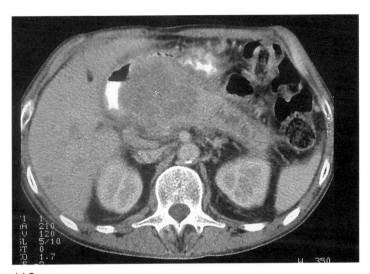

118. This is a contrast-enhanced abdominal CT scan of a patient who was admitted with acute upper abdominal and back pain.

a. Describe the abnormality.
b. Suggest a diagnosis and give two causes.
c. Outline treatment.

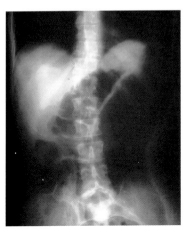

119. This abdominal X-ray is of a 29-year-old man with ulcerative colitis who developed abdominal pain and distension.

a. What complication has occurred?
b. Outline treatment.

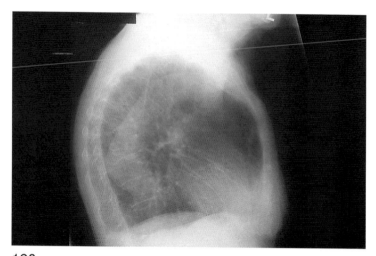

120. This lateral chest X-ray is of a 74-year-old woman with chronic back pain.

a. Describe the abnormality.
b. What condition does this patient have?
c. Give three predisposing causes.

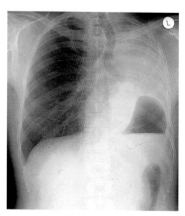

121. This is a chest X-ray of a 47-year-old smoker.

a. Describe the abnormalities.
b. Give a differential diagnosis.
c. What further investigations may be indicated?

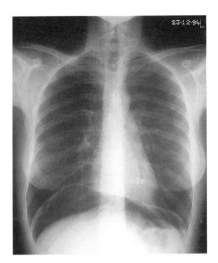

122. This is a chest X-ray of a 24-year-old woman with abdominal pain.

a. Describe the abnormality.
b. Give a differential diagnosis.
c. What treatment is indicated?

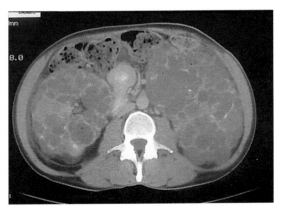

123. This is an abdominal CT scan of a 31-year-old woman.

a. What is the diagnosis and what is the inheritance?
b. Give an associated condition.
c. What complications may occur?

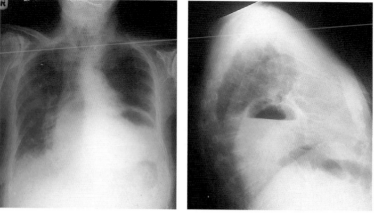

A   B

124. These X-rays are from an 82-year-old woman.

a. Describe the abnormality and suggest a diagnosis.

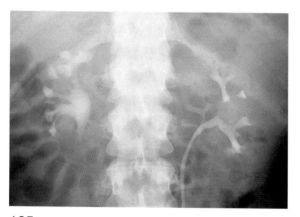

125. This intravenous urogram is from a 29-year-old woman who was referred to the medical outpatients department following the incidental discovery of proteinuria.

a. Describe the abnormality.
b. Outline management.

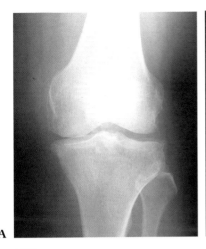

A

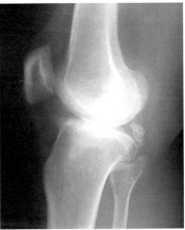

B

126. These right knee X-rays are of a 60-year-old man who complains of recurrent pain in, and swelling of, his knee.

a. Describe the abnormality.
b. Suggest a diagnosis.
c. What other joint symptoms may he have?
d. What investigation is indicated?

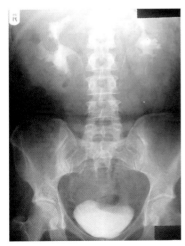

127. This intravenous urogram is from a 50-year-old lady.

a. Describe the abnormality and suggest the likely diagnosis.
b. Give five modes of presentation.
c. Outline management.

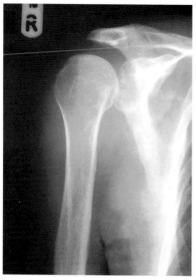

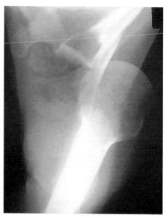

B

A

128. **This known epileptic had a painful shoulder following a grand mal fit.**

a. What do his AP and axial views demonstrate?
b. What is the immediate management?

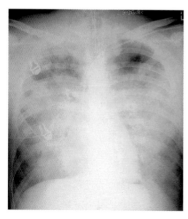

129. **This chest X-ray is from a 34-year-old man.**

a. Describe the abnormalities.
b. Suggest a clinical diagnosis.
c. Give four underlying causes.

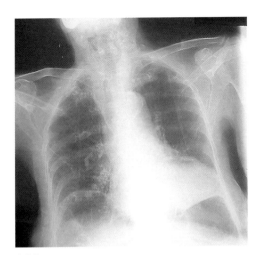

130. This is a chest X-ray of an 84-year-old woman with intermittent right upper quadrant discomfort.

a. Are the lung fields normal?
b. What is the name for the the unusual pattern of bowel gas distribution?
c. What further investigations are required?

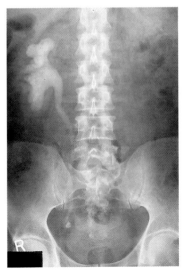

131. This is a delayed (2 hour) film from an intravenous urogram of a 59-year-old man who is oliguric and who has a long history of renal calculi.

a. Describe the abnormality.
b. What further investigations and treatment should be undertaken?

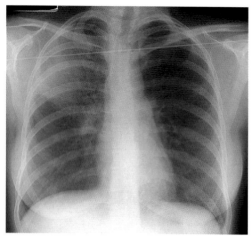

A

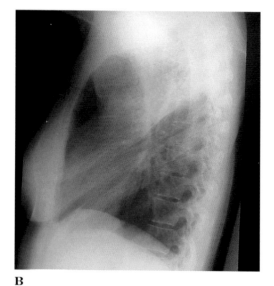

B

132. **These X-rays are of a 33-year-old woman.**

a. Describe the abnormality and give the diagnosis.

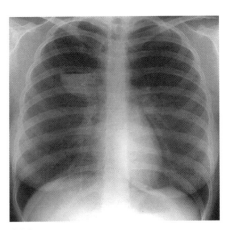

133. This chest X-ray is of a 26-year-old woman with copious purulent sputum and swinging fever.

a. Describe the abnormality.
b. Give three predisposing conditions.

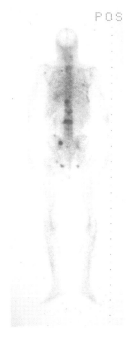

POS

134. This isotope bone scan is from a 68-year-old man.

a. What is demonstrated?
b. Suggest a cause.
c. Suggest two useful investigations.

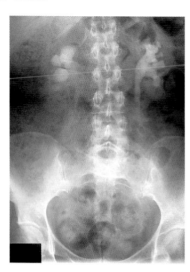

135. This intravenous urogram is from a 52-year-old woman with a 2 year history of mid-back pain and weight loss.

a. Describe the abnormality.
b. Give a differential diagnosis.
c. What further investigations are indicated?

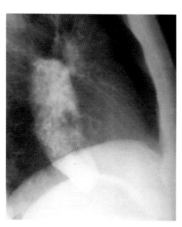

136. This barium swallow is from a 43-year-old woman with a long history of dysphagia.

a. Describe the abnormality.
b. What is the diagnosis and what other symptoms might she complain of?
c. Outline management.
d. What are the potential complications?

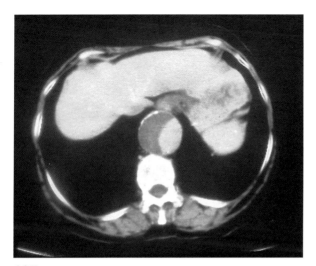

137. This is a contrast-enhanced thoracic CT scan of a patient who presented to the casualty department with severe acute chest pain.

a. What is the diagnosis?
b. Describe the abnormality.
c. What physical signs should be sought?
d. What treatment is indicated?

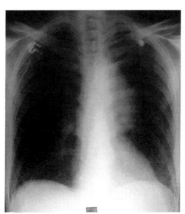

138. This chest X-ray is of a 58-year-old smoker who has had numerous chest infections over the preceding winter.

a. Describe the abnormality.
b. What is the differential diagnosis?

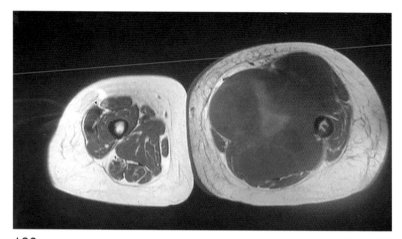

139. This MRI scan is of an 80-year-old woman who has rapidly developed a swollen left thigh.

a. Describe the abnormality and suggest a diagnosis.

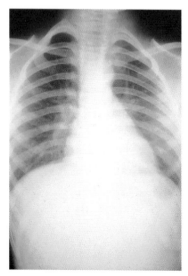

140. This chest X-ray is of a 34-year-old man who complains of weakness of his left hand together with paraesthesia affecting the ulnar border of his forearm.

a. What is the diagnosis?
b. What is the cause of his symptoms?
c. What other symptoms might he complain of?

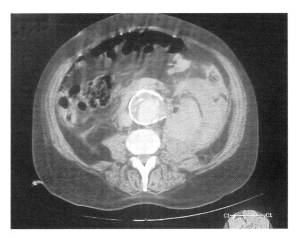

A

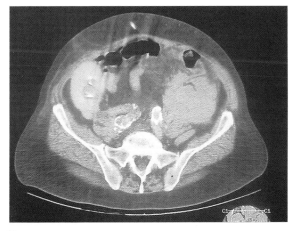

B

141. These contrast-enhanced abdominal and pelvic CT scans are of a 63-year-old man who was admitted with sudden onset of left-sided abdominal pain. The haemoglobin fell from 11.6 to 7.9 g/dl without obvious gastrointestinal haemorrhage.

a. Describe the abnormality.
b. Suggest two diagnoses.
b. Outline treatment.

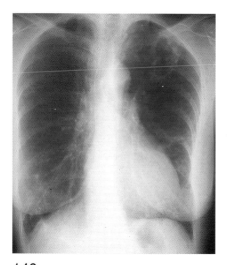

142. **This chest X-ray is of a 67-year-old smoker with recurrent haemoptysis.**

a. Describe the abnormality.
b. What is the most likely diagnosis?

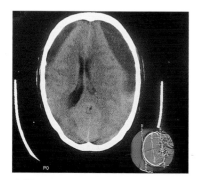

143. **This is a CT brain scan of a 62-year-old diabetic man who has become increasingly confused over several weeks.**

a. Describe the abnormality.
b. Suggest a predisposing cause.
c. What treatment is indicated?

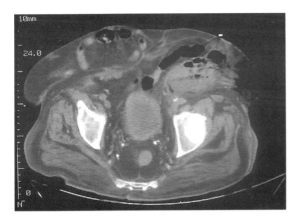

144. This is a pelvic CT scan of a 48-year-old diabetic man who has recently received a left renal transplant and who has been admitted with a high fever and rigors.

a. Describe the abnormality.
b. Suggest a diagnosis.
c. What treatment is indicated?

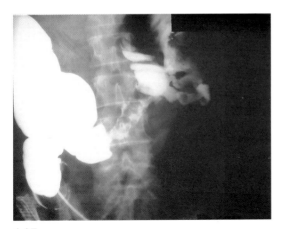

145. This barium study is from a 63-year-old man who has had a defunctioning caecostomy for large bowel obstruction.

a. Describe the abnormality.
b. How else may this condtion present?
c. What treatment is indicated?

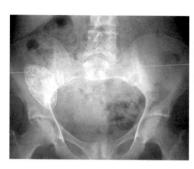

146. This abdominal X-ray is of a 58-year-old woman who is on maintenance haemodialysis.

a. Describe the abnormality.
b. Suggest a cause.

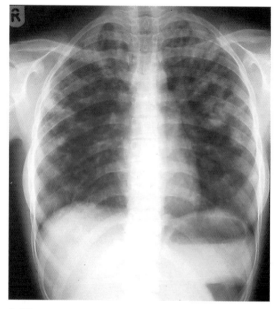

147. This is a chest X-ray of a previously well 16-year-old Asian woman who complains of a chronic cough and weight loss.

a. Describe the abnormality.
b. What is the most likely diagnosis?
c. Give two other causes.
d. What further investigations are required?

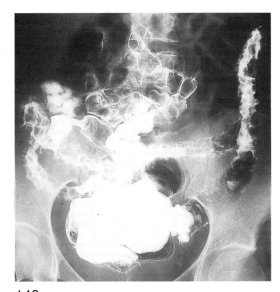

148. This barium meal and follow-through is from a 45-year-old woman who has had a previous right hemicolectomy. She has recently developed intermittent abdominal pain.

a. Describe the abnormality.
b. Suggest a diagnosis.
c. Give three potential complications.

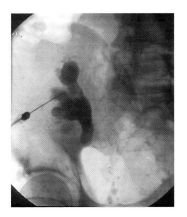

149. This antegrade pyelogram is from a 60-year-old renal transplant patient with deteriorating renal function.

a. Describe the abnormality.
b. Suggest a cause.
c. What treatment can be offered?

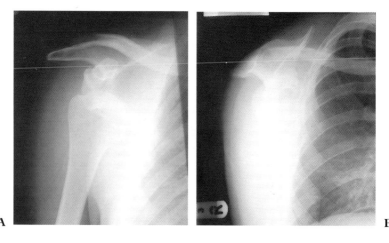

A   B

150. This young man injured his shoulder playing rugby. All movements were reduced in range and painful.

a. What is the injury?
b. What is the management?

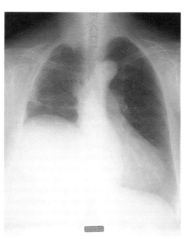

151. This is a routine chest X-ray of an asymptomatic 74-year-old woman.

a. Describe the abnormalities.
b. What condition has this patient had?
c. What treatment has been given in the past?

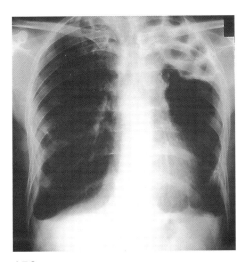

152. This chest X-ray is of a 76-year-old man.

a. Describe the abnormality.
b. What condition has this patient had and what treatment has been given?

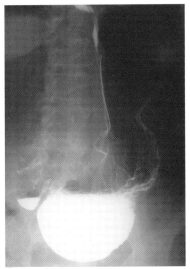

153. This barium swallow is from a 59-year-old woman with dyspepsia.

a. Describe the abnormality.
b. Outline management.

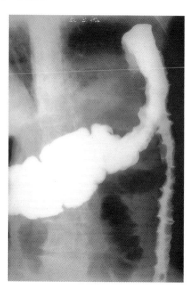

154. This is a barium enema film on an elderly lady presenting with acute and marked rectal bleeding.

a. What does this barium enema film show?
b. What is the clinical management?
c. What are the possible complications?

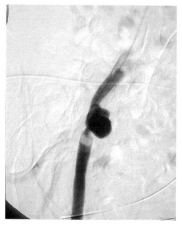

155. This digital subtraction arteriogram of the right external iliac artery (via left femoral approach) was performed in a 38-year-old man who was recovering from a severe septicaemia when he developed a painful blotchy skin rash over his right foot.

a. Describe the abnormality.
b. What is the most likely diagnosis?
c. What is the cause of the rash?
d. What treatment is indicated?

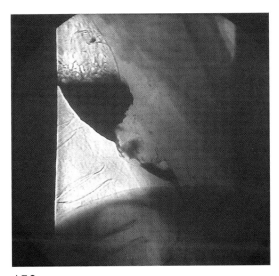

156. This barium swallow is from a 69-year-old lady with recent onset dysphagia.

a. Describe the abnormality.
b. What is the diagnosis?
c. Outline management.

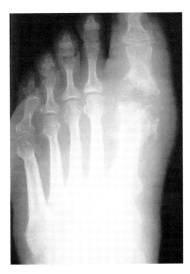

157. This left foot X-ray is from a 50-year-old man.

a. Describe the abnormality.
b. Suggest a diagnosis.
c. What treatment is available?

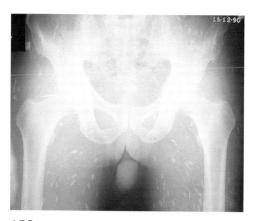

158. This X-ray is from a 19-year-old Indian student who was admitted to hospital following an epileptic fit.

a. Describe the abnormality.
b. What condition has this patient had?
c. What further investigation is required?
d. What treatment is indicated?

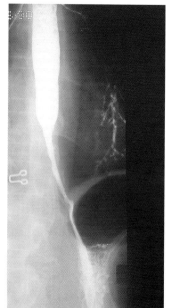

159. This barium swallow is from a 50-year-old lady with long-standing dyspepsia.

a. Describe the abnormality and suggest a diagnosis.
b. Outline management.

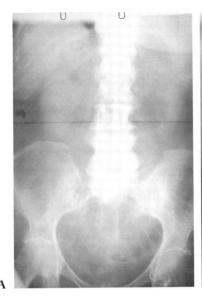

A

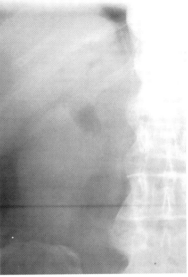

B

160. This elderly lady was admitted in an acutely unwell state with abdominal pains and vomiting.

a. What do this supine abdominal X-ray and the close-up of the right upper quadrant show?
b. What is the diagnosis?

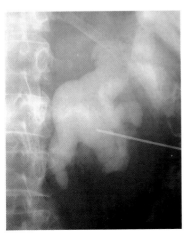

161. This antegrade pyelogram is from a 53-year-old woman who was admitted to hospital with a fever and left loin pain.

a. Describe the abnormality.
b. What treatment is required?

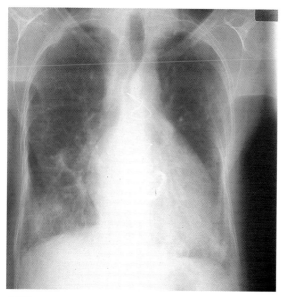

162. This is a chest X-ray of a 60-year-old lady.

a. What surgical procedure has been performed previously?
b. What physical signs may be present?
c. What advice should she have been given?

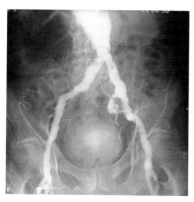

163. This arteriogram was performed in a 67-year-old man with renal impairment.

a. Describe the abnormalities.
b. Suggest a cause for the renal impairment.
c. What symptoms might the patient complain of?

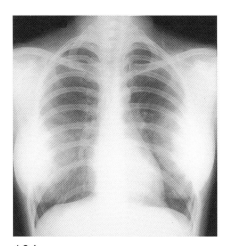

164. This chest X-ray is of a 30-year-old woman.

a. Describe the abnormality.
b. What surgical procedure has been performed?

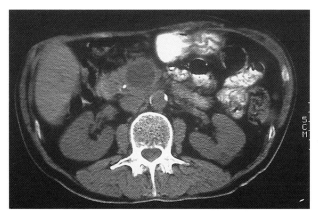

165. This is an abdominal CT scan of a 58-year-old man who presented with weight loss and abdominal pain.

a. Describe the abnormality.
b. Suggest a diagnosis.
c. What treatment is available?

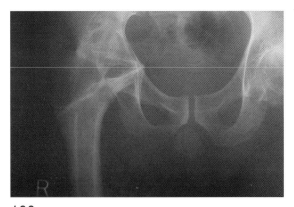

166. **This pelvic X-ray is of a 63-year-old man who had tuberculosis of the right hip in 1947.**

a. What treatment was performed for the tuberculosis?
b. What complication has arisen from this?

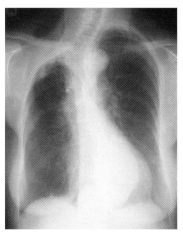

167. **This chest X-ray is from a 60-year-old woman.**

a. Describe the abnormalities.
b. What condition has this patient had?
c. What treatment has been given and why?

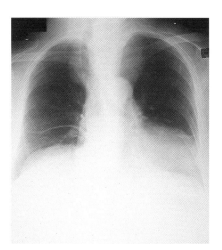

168. This is a chest X-ray of a 78-year-old lady who complains of recent onset 'asthma'.

a. Describe the mediastinal abnormality.
b. Suggest a cause.
c. What further investigations are indicated?
d. What treatment is required?

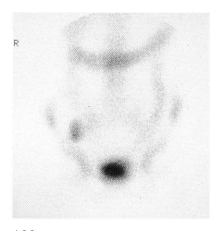

169. This white cell scan is of a 19-year-old man.

a. Describe the abnormality.
b. Suggest a cause.

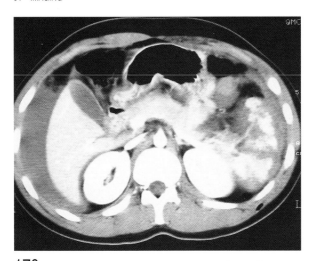

170. This contrast-enhanced abdominal CT scan is of a
40-year-old man who was admitted to hospital in a shocked state
and complaining of abdominal pain after being involved in a
road traffic accident.

a. Describe the abnormality.
b. Outline treatment.

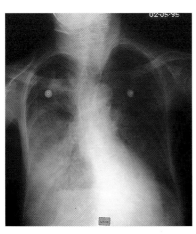

171. This chest X-ray is of an
85-year-old woman who was
admitted to hospital unable to
cope at home.

a. Describe the abnormality.
b. Outline the investigations and
management.

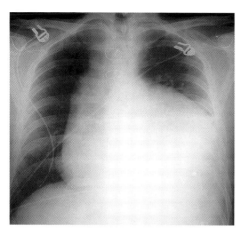

A

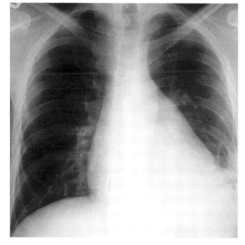

B

172. **(A) is a chest X-ray of a 64-year-old man who was admitted to hospital feeling generally unwell. (B) is a follow-up chest X-ray. He had undergone coronary artery bypass grafting 9 years previously.**

a. Describe the abnormalities.
b. What is the diagnosis and what treatment has been given?
c. Give three causes.

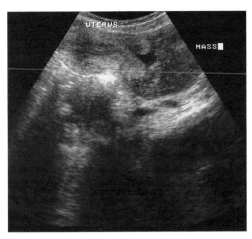

A

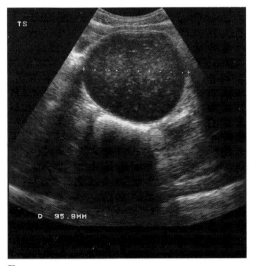

B

173. This 17-year-old girl was referred by her GP for an urgent pelvic ultrasound. She had primary amenorrhoea and a pelvic mass arising from the pelvic cavity.

a. What diagnosis should be considered clinically?
b. What does the ultrasound scan show?
c. What is the management?

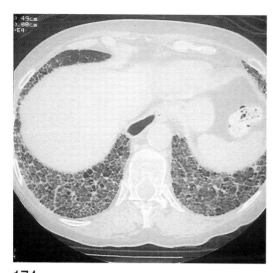

174. This is a high-resolution lung CT scan of a 67-year-old man with progressive dyspnoea on exertion.

a. Describe the abnormality.
b. What is the diagnosis?
c. Give three causes.
d. What physical signs may be present?

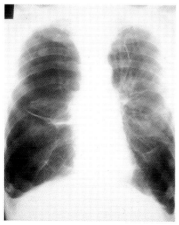

175. This chest X-ray is of a 39-year-old man who requires domiciliary oxygen.

a. Describe the abnormalities.
b. Suggest a diagnosis.
c. What is the inheritance of the condition?
d. What other organ may be adveresly affected?
e. What treatment is available?

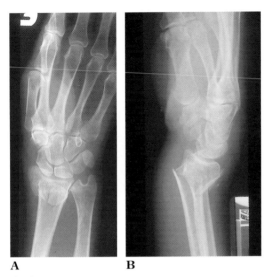

A B

176. These X-rays are of a 69-year-old woman who fell in her garden.

a. Describe the abnormality.
b. What is the diagnosis?
c. Give two predisposing conditions.

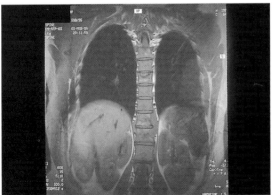

177. This MRI scan is of a 24-year-old Asian woman who has a 6 month history of lower dorsal back pain. She has a low grade fever and a raised erythrocyte sedimentation rate (ESR) of 86 mm/h.

a. Describe the abnormality and suggest a diagnosis.

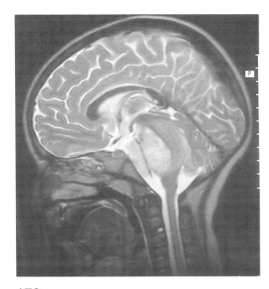

178. **This sagittal midline T2 weighted MRI scan (i.e. CSF appears white) is of a 6-year-old girl with a history of headaches and ataxia.**

a. Describe the abnormality and suggest a diagnosis.

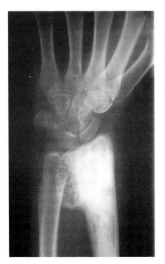

179. **This 16-year-old girl attended casualty with a painful wrist after a relatively trivial injury.**

a. What does the plain film show?
b. What is the management?

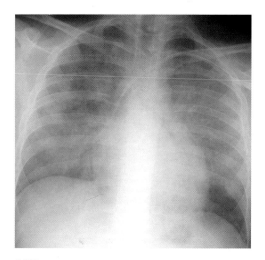

180. This chest X-ray is of an 18-year-old man who has recently been heavily immunosuppressed for a crescentic glomerulonephritis. He is unwell, febrile and markedly hypoxic.

a. Describe the abnormality.
b. Suggest a diagnosis and outline management.

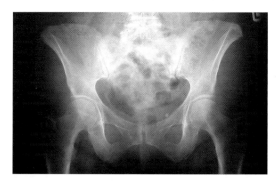

181. This pelvic X-ray is of an asymptomatic 76-year-old woman.

a. Describe the abnormality.
b. What condition does this patient have?
c. What blood test will be abnormal?
d. Give three possible complications.

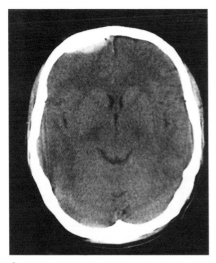

A

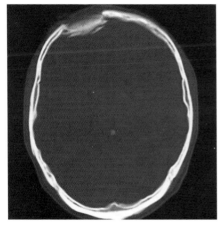

B

182. These two CT head images are of a man who sustained a direct focal head injury, having been hit with a heavy object. He was fully conscious on arrival at hospital.

a. Describe the abnormality on each of the images.
b. What is the immediate management?
c. What are the possible long-term complications of such an injury?

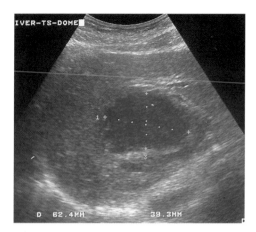

183. This is a liver ultrasound examination of a 66-year-old man who presented with a persistent fever.

a. Describe the abnormality.
b. Give a differential diagnosis.

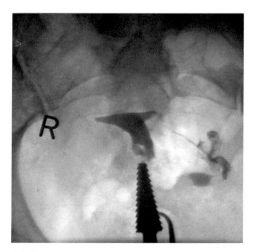

184. a. What is this investigation and what does it show?
   b. Give two causes of this appearance.

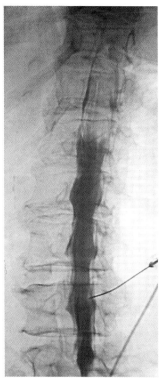 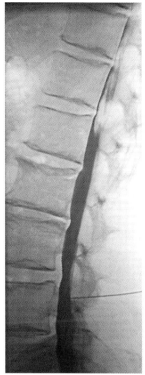

A   B

185. This myelogram was performed in a 69-year-old who complains of difficulty in walking.

a. What does it show?
b. Suggest a diagnosis.

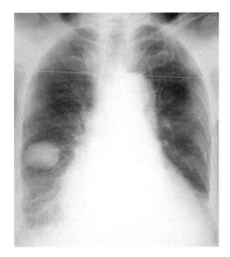

A

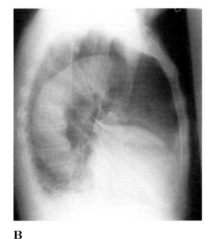

B

186. These X-rays are of a 69-year-old man.

a. Describe the abnormality and suggest a diagnosis.
b. What treatment is indicated?

Answers

1.   a. There is a linear shadow extending from the left hilum along the left heart border.
    b. Pneumopericardium.

2.   a. Horner's syndrome consists of a partial ptosis, a sunken eye (enophthalmos) and a constricted pupil (miosis), together with a lack of sweating (anhidrosis) on the affected side of the face.
    b. The right breast shadow is absent and, as a result, the right lower zone is more radiolucent than the left lower zone. There is ill-defined peripheral shadowing in the right upper zone.
    c. The most likely diagnosis is recurrent carcinoma of the breast with neoplastic infiltration of the cervical sympathetic chain.

3.   a. Scan (A) reveals a high density mass with mainly peripheral calcification which subsequently shows strong homogenous enhancement with contrast. There is relatively little vasogenic oedema adjacent to the mass.
    b. Meningioma (of the sphenoid wing).
    c. Neurosurgery.

4.   a. This is a renal angiogram.
    b. There is a proximal right renal artery stenosis. The right kidney is considerably smaller than the normally perfused left kidney, indicating long standing ischaemia.
    c. Hypertension.
    d. Percutaneous balloon angioplasty is the treatment of choice.

5.   a. The left kidney is non-visualised while the right kidney is normal.
    b. The following investigations are indicated:
- ultrasound or CT scan to assess whether the left kidney is absent or small and non-functioning
- routine immunological tests including immunoglobulins, Bence–Jones protein, autoantibody screen, etc.
- flexible cystoscopy in order to exclude a bladder lesion.

    Obviously a renal biopsy should not be performed in a patient with a single kidney unless it is imperative to obtain a diagnosis, in which case one should consider performing an open 'surgical' biopsy to ensure haemostasis.

6.
a. There are multiple rounded opacities of varying size throughout both lung fields. This appearance is consistent with multiple metastases.
b. The primary tumour most commonly arises from the lung, breast, colon, thyroid or testes.
c. Such advanced disease is almost always incurable, although palliative chemotherapy may be of benefit in some cases.

7.
a. There are marked honeycomb changes affecting the right middle lobe.
b. Cystic bronchiectasis.
c. Causes include:
   • previous infections, especially measles or 'whooping cough'
   • bronchial obstruction, e.g. foreign body
   • immunodeficiency states, e.g. hypogammaglobulinaemia or chronic granulomatous disease
   • immotile cilia syndrome
   • cystic fibrosis.
d. Patients may develop:
   • acute infective exacerbations with pneumonia and pleurisy
   • haemoptysis, which can be torrential
   • systemic amyloidosis
   • brain abscess.

8.
a. There is a low attenuation mass projecting from the cortex of the left kidney.
b. Left hypernephroma.
c. Patients may present with:
   • macroscopic haematuria (the majority of patients)
   • hypercalcaemia secondary to the production of ectopic parathormone-like substance by the tumour or bone metastases
   • constitutional upset including flank pain (with palpable mass if large tumour), weight loss, pyrexia of unknown origin, elevated ESR, etc.
   • recent onset left-sided varicocoele if the left testicular vein is involved.

9.
a. There is contrast within the right iliac vein and inferior vena cava, while some contrast is being excreted by the kidneys. A filling defect is present within the iliac vein and inferior vena cava, representing thrombus. A 'bird's nest' filter has been positioned within the inferior vena cava.
b. This procedure may be of great benefit in patients who have developed significant venous thrombosis and who are therefore at risk of a life-threatening pulmonary embolus, but in whom anticoagulation with heparin or warfarin is very

hazardous, e.g. those with a recent cerebral haemorrhage, ongoing gastrointestinal bleeding, etc.

10.
 a. There is bilateral upper zone fibrosis together with a mass in the left upper zone which has a crescent of air superiorly.
 b. A mycetoma or 'fungus ball' (usually an aspergilloma) within a pre-existing cavity, e.g. previous tuberculosis.
 c. Serum precipitins to *Aspergillus fumigatus* are usually high, while the organism may be cultured from the sputum.
 d. Most patients are asymptomatic, but surgical excision may be required for severe or recurrent haemoptysis.

11.
 a. There is a very large abdominal aortic aneurysm, with contrast within the central lumen which is surrounded by mural thrombus. Calcification is evident in the wall of the aorta. There is erosion of the anterior aspect of the adjacent vertebrae.
 b. Patients may complain of:
  • other symptoms of peripheral vascular disease such as intermittent claudication
  • back pain or abdominal discomfort
  • peripheral embolisation to the lower limbs.
 c. Predisposing factors include:
  • hypertension
  • cigarette smoking
  • metabolic disorders such as hyperlipidaemia and diabetes mellitus.
 d. Treatment may be conservative if the patient is medically unfit. Graft replacement of the diseased segment is the standard surgical option, while endovascular procedures are under development.

12.
 a. There is a large left pleural effusion.
 b. The most likely diagnoses in a man of this age are:
  • primary bronchial carcinoma
  • metastatic tumour or, more rarely, lymphoma
  • tuberculosis.
 c. Pleural biopsy and aspiration of pleural fluid (cytology, protein, glucose and microbiological culture for mycobacterium tuberculosis), sputum cytology and culture, and bronchoscopy.

13.
 a. There is air within the upper portion of the right orbit— 'orbital emphysema'.
 b. This indicates that the patient has sustained a fracture involving the paranasal sinuses. The patient should be assessed by an ophthalmic or maxillofacial department to

ensure there are no significant visual problems (caused by mechanical trapping of an extraocular muscle).

14.
a. There is an opacity overlying the left renal outline which represents a staghorn calculus.
b. Staghorn calculi are composed of magnesium ammonium phosphate plus calcium and are associated with infection of the urinary tract with 'urea-splitting' organisms, e.g. *Proteus mirabilis*.
c. Treatment available includes the following:
  - Open surgery to remove the stone (pyelolithotomy) is often required for large staghorn calculi as in this case.
  - Smaller stones can be removed by percutaneous nephrolithotomy, or they can be fragmented using lithotripsy.
  - A high fluid intake and rigorous detection and treatment of urinary tract infections, including antibiotic prophylaxis, may prevent further stone formation.

15.
a. There is linear calcification between the articular surfaces.
b. Chondrocalcinosis of the menisci and calcium pyrophosphate arthropathy (pseudogout).
c. Associated conditions include:
  - haemachromatosis
  - primary hyperparathyroidism
  - hypothyroidism
  - acromegaly
  - hypophosphataemia.
d. Treatment is symptomatic and includes:
  - rest and other simple physical measures
  - analgesics and non-steroidal anti-inflammatory drugs may be helpful
  - aspiration of acutely inflamed joints (must exclude a septic arthritis), together with intra-articular steroid injection.

16.
a. (A) shows a Swan–Ganz catheter (it is far too long to be a central venous catheter) which has been passed down the inferior vena cava into the hepatic vein. In (B), a chest drain has inadvertently been inserted below the left hemidiaphragm. In (C), a nasogastric tube has been passed into the right main bronchus despite the presence of a tracheostomy. In (D), there is a complete left pneumothorax following the insertion of a permanent pacemaker.

17.
a. There is extensive right-sided pleural thickening extending onto the mediastinal reflection.
b. Malignant mesothelioma.

c. Exposure to asbestos.

d. Physical signs include clubbing and hypertrophic pulmonary osteopathy.

e. Chemotherapy and radiotherapy are of limited use in this disease. Surgery may be of benefit in occasional selected cases.

18.

a. The striking abnormality is marked dilatation of the large bowel, particularly affecting the rectum. There has also been a right hemiarthroplasty, and a calcified lymph node is evident within the pelvis.

b. Pseudo-obstruction, since gas is visible throughout the large bowel including the rectum.

c. Passage of a flatus tube may be beneficial.

19.

a. There is a localised bulge on the left heart border.

b. Left ventricular aneurysm.

c. Patients may present with:
   - cardiac failure
   - ventricular dysrhythmias
   - arterial embolisation from thrombus within the aneurysm
   - persistent ST segment elevation on the electrocardiograph.

d. Treatment may include:
   - Surgical excision of the aneurysm
   - anticoagulation, in view of the risk of systemic embolisation
   - pharmacological treatment of dysrhythmias.

20.

a. There is cardiomegaly with splaying of the carina, indicating dilatation of the left atrium. There is egg shell calcification evident, presumably within atrial mural thrombus. This patient has mitral valve disease and may well benefit from anticoagulation with warfarin in order to reduce the probability of systemic embolisation.

21.

a. There is blood within the ventricles and around the cerebral sulci.

b. Extensive subarachnoid haemorrhage. The commonest cause is a ruptured berry aneurysm, while arteriovenous malformations are less common. There are two possible reasons for her hypoxia:
   - neurogenic pulmonary oedema
   - extensive aspiration of stomach contents.

c. Treatment consists of:
   - intravenous nimodipine, which reduces vasospasm
   - a ventricular shunt may be inserted if the patient develops hydrocephalus

- some aneurysms may be amenable to surgical clipping (cerebral angiography needed when patient is stable)
- neurogenic pulmonary oedema may be treated with oxygen and diuretics, but ventilation may be required
- aspiration pneumonia requires broad-spectrum antibiotics with or without ventilation.

22.
a. The colon is narrowed and is gas-filled with no faecal residue. This is a 'hosepipe colon'.
b. Long-standing ulcerative colitis.
c. Complications of ulcerative colitis include:
- haemorrhage, toxic dilatation and perforation
- carcinoma of the colon
- arthritis, including sacroiliitis, ankylosing spondylitis or an asymmetrical polyarthropathy typically affecting large joints
- sclerosing cholangitis
- systemic amyloidosis may occur rarely.

23.
a. The ribs are 'flat' and there is a marked scoliolis.
b. Respiratory failure, with nocturnal hypoxia, hypercapnia and secondary right heart failure resulting from a restrictive kyphoscoliosis.
c. Arterial blood gases to assess the degree of hypoxia and hypercapnia, together with a sleep study to document nocturnal hypoxia.
d. Recently, nocturnal nasal intermittent positive pressure ventilation (NIPPV) has been used with some success. Right-sided heart failure, if present, may be treated with diuretics, while polycythaemia requires venesection.

24.
a. There is a small cluster of radio-opaque gallstones in the right upper quadrant as well as osteoarthritic changes affecting the hip joints and lumbar vertebrae. The history is suggestive of biliary colic.
b. Other complications include:
- acute or chronic cholecystitis
- acute pancreatitis
- obstructive jaundice which can result in an ascending cholangitis if complicated by infection
- gallstone ileus may occur if the stone erodes through the gallbladder wall into the small bowel usually impacting at the terminal ileum.
c. Acute episodes of biliary colic are managed conservatively with analgesia and anti-emetics. An open or laparoscopic cholecystectomy is indicated for recurrent episodes.

25.
a. There is a large intracerebral bleed into the left cerebral hemisphere, with blood evident within the ventricles and a midline shift from left to right secondary to the mass effect.
b. Predisposing conditions include:
- hypertension
- atheromatous disease
- bleeding disorders or over-anticoagulation with warfarin.

26.
a. There is extensive right-sided pleural thickening and calcification, with associated apical pleural thickening and marked loss of volume of the right lung. The appearance is typical of previous pulmonary tuberculosis and a tuberculous empyema. An alternative would be any cause leading to a haemothorax.

27.
a. The patient has had a Starr–Edwards aortic valve replacement.
b. Possible indications for surgery include:
- severe aortic stenosis, e.g. of a congenital bicuspid valve
- progressive aortic incompetence
- infective endocarditis.
c. Complications include:
- infection
- complications arising from the necessary anticoagulation with warfarin, such as gastrointestinal bleeding
- haemolysis
- thrombosis of the valve, which can occur if the INR is too low.
d. Diastole.

28.
a. There is a raised mucosal and ulcerated mass on the posterior aspect of the body of the stomach (confirmed on other projections). The appearances suggest malignant transformation at the site of a chronic gastric ulcer.
b. Endoscopic biopsy. If confirmed to be malignant, a staging ultrasound scan or CT scan should be performed to assess for liver deposits.

29.
a. There is consolidation of the left lingula.
b. This radiological picture may result from infection with many organisms which can cause a primary pneumonic illness, including *Streptococcus pneumoniae* and *Haemophilus influenzae*, as well as the organisms causing the 'atypical' pneumonias. These include *Mycoplasma pneumoniae*, *Legionella pneumophila*, *Chlamydia pneumoniae* and *Ch. psittaci*. The latter organism is contracted from infected birds, such as parrots, and should be strongly considered in this patient.

    c. Treatment of primary pneumonias varies slightly from place to place depending on the local antibiotic sensitivities of the common pathogens, but amoxycillin/cefuroxime with erythromycin will be adequate in most patients. This patient should also receive tetracycline, in view of his occupation, until the cause of the infection has been elucidated.

30.
    a. There are minor spondylotic changes affecting the spine, but bilateral curvilinear calcification is evident, representing a large abdominal aortic aneurysm which is the most likely cause of his symptoms.

    b. This patient has a large symptomatic abdominal aortic aneurysm and requires urgent referral to a vascular surgeon in order to assess whether he is fit for interventional surgery.

31.
    a. There is a large mass in the left midzone.

    b. Primary bronchial neoplasm.

    c. Hypercalcaemia (bony metastases or release of ectopic PTH-like substance), deranged liver functions tests (secondary spread), hypoalbuminaemia and normochromic anaemia.

    d. Either bronchoscopy or CT-guided needle biopsy is required to obtain a histological diagnosis.

    e. Surgery (if no imaging evidence of metastases and if the patient is medically fit) or chemotherapy with or without radiotherapy.

32.
    a. There are multiple air–fluid levels within the centrally located small bowel, and there is an absence of air from the large bowel indicating small bowel obstruction.

    b. Physical signs present may include:
- abdominal distension
- 'tinkling' active bowel sounds.

    c. Possible causes include:
- adhesions from previous surgery
- an incarcerated or strangulated external (or rarely internal) hernia
- Crohn's disease
- intra-abdominal or pelvic malignancy.

    d. Treatment consists of:
- passage of a nasogastric tube
- intravenous fluids and analgesia
- surgery, if the obstruction does not resolve with conservative management or if there are signs of peritonism (suggesting strangulated ischaemic bowel).

33.
    a. There is a calcified linear plaque on the left diaphragm which is the result of previous asbestos exposure.

34.

a. There is dextrocardia. Note that the gastric air bubble is normally situated, thereby excluding a situs inversus.

b. The ECG would show right axis deviation with loss of R waves across the chest leads.

c. Enquiries should be made regarding symptoms suggesting associated bronchiectasis and sinus disease (Kartagener's syndrome).

35.

a. The left hemithorax is radiolucent and there is gross mediastinal shift to the right, indicating a left tension pneumothorax.

b. The diagnosis of a tension pneumothorax is clinical, and treatment should be instituted before obtaining radiological confirmation of the diagnosis, i.e. a cannula should be inserted into the affected side followed by insertion of an underwater seal chest drain.

36.

a. There is a large well-defined lesion in the right lobe of the liver with a central area of low attenuation.

b. Hepatoma.

c. Previous hepatitis B infection or cirrhosis of any aetiology.

d. Surgical resection may be curative if the tumour is confined to one lobe. Chemotherapy is disappointing while radiotherapy does not help. The tumour marker alpha fetoprotein may be of use in monitoring response to therapy. Intra-arterial infusion of cytotoxic agents with or without tumour embolisation may occasionally be indicated.

37.

a. There is a transonic mass at the upper pole of a normal right testis. This is a simple epididymal cyst.

b. The patient should be reassured that there is no evidence of a malignant lesion. Surgery should be reserved for patients who have discomfort or in whom the cysts are multiple and increase in size.

38.

a. The patient has a tracheostomy in situ and has been ventilated for respiratory failure consequent upon the acute infection. The lungs are hyperinflated (greater than six anterior ribs seen above the diaphragm in the mid-clavicular line) with flat ribs and diaphragm and reduced peripheral vascular markings. A left mastectomy has been performed previously.

b. Emphysema.

c. Smoking, although alpha-1-antitrypsin deficiency is a possible though rare cause.

d. Physical signs include:
   - reduced crico-sternal distance and chest expansion

- quiet breath sounds
- peripheral and central cyanosis.

39.
a. There is a large region of increased radiolucency in the left hemithorax with an absence of lung markings.
b. Left pneumothorax.
c. Spontaneous (especially in tall thin men), blunt or penetrating chest injuries, or iatrogenic (e.g. attempted insertion of central line).
d. Insertion of an underwater seal chest drain.

40.
a. There is extensive diverticulosis of the sigmoid colon.
b. Approximately 30% of the population has diverticulosis by the age of 60 years and therefore many individuals have no symptoms. However, complications include:
- painless rectal bleeding which can be severe and can require blood transfusion or even surgery
- intermittent left iliac fossa discomfort
- diverticulitis which may result in perforation and faecal peritonitis
- fistulae to the bladder or vagina
- stricture formation following previous inflammation.
c. Management consists of the following:
- high fibre diet
- anti-spasmodic agents
- diverticulitis usually settles with intravenous fluids and antibiotics, while fistulae, perforation etc. require surgery.

41.
a. There is a normal right kidney and a duplex left kidney.
b. No.
c. A patient of this age with haematuria merits a cystoscopy in order to exclude a bladder neoplasm.

42.
a. There is speckled calcification overlying the 12th thoracic vertebral body.
b. Chronic pancreatitis.
c. Causes include:
- chronic alcohol abuse
- cystic fibrosis
- long-standing obstruction to the pancreatic duct.
d. Treatment consists of the following:
- pancreatic enzyme supplements with meals
- abstinence from alcohol
- patients may require treatment for resultant diabetes mellitus
- surgery may be indicated if pain is severe and unremitting.

43.
a. There are multiple lytic metastatic deposits, particularly in the pubic rami. No pathological fracture is evident.

b. Tumours that commonly metastasise to bones include carcinoma of the stomach, colon, thyroid, lung and breast (in women).

c. Abnormalities on routine blood tests include:
- anaemia, while the blood film may show a leucoerythroblastic picture
- biochemical tests may reveal hyponatraemia, hypercalcaemia and deranged liver function tests.

44.
a. Numerous septal lines (Kerley B lines) are evident. These are 1–3 cm long; they extend from, and are perpendicular to, the pleural surface; and they are visible interlobular lymphatics.

b. Causes include:
- pulmonary venous hypertension, e.g. left ventricular failure or mitral stenosis
- obstruction of the lymphatic system, e.g. lymphangitis carcinomatosa.

45.
a. There is marked disorganisation of the tarsal bones.

b. This is a Charcot or neuropathic joint and results from repeated minor trauma due to a severe neuropathy. Causes include:
- diabetes mellitus
- syringomyelia
- leprosy and syphilis, which are important causes worldwide.

46.
a. There is marked cardiomegaly with prominent upper lobe veins but no other features of heart failure. This appearance suggests a cardiomyopathy, in this case secondary to ethanol.

b. Physical signs may include:
- displaced apex beat
- low volume pulse
- stigmata of chronic liver disease, including jaundice, leuchonychia, clubbing, Dupuytren's contracture, spider naevi, hepatomegaly, splenomegaly, ascites or a glove-and-stocking neuropathy.

c. Abstinence from alcohol, vitamin B supplementation if indicated, together with conventional treatment for cardiac failure (diuretics, angiotensin-converting enzyme inhibitors and vasodilators).

47.
a. There is a large, predominantly cystic, ovoid lesion with an eccentrically placed solid nodular component. The

appearance is highly suspicious of a malignant ovarian tumour.

b. Treatment consists of surgery, and possibly chemotherapy and radiotherapy depending on the stage of the tumour.

48.
a. There is a mature infarct in the left occipital cortex with associated ballooning of the posterior horn of the lateral ventricle. In addition, there are also multiple small lacunar infarcts and global cerebral atrophy with general sulci widening.

b. Multiple infarcts can be the result of cerebral atheromatous disease or multiple embolic phenomena.

49.
a. There is fusion of the sacroiliac joints together with ankylosis of the lumbar vertebrae.

b. Ankylosing spondylitis.

c. Associations include inflammatory bowel disease and psoriasis.

50.
a. There is an accumulation of labelled white cells below the liver.

b. The most likely cause is a subhepatic abscess.

c. Drainage and microbiological culture of the pus are mandatory, followed by treatment with appropriate antibiotics.

51.
a. Abnormalities include:
  - generalised osteopaenia
  - subluxation of the metacarpophalangeal joints
  - carpal fusion
  - ulnar deviation.

b. This radiological appearance can be found in rheumatoid arthritis or psoriatic arthropathy.

c. Psoriasis can be associated with a severe symmetrical deforming arthropathy identical to rheumatoid arthritis, but the presence of skin disease (which may be mild) and nail pitting distinguishes it from rheumatoid arthritis which may be associated with rheumatoid nodules.

52.
a. Percutaneous transhepatic cholangiography (PTC).

b. There is marked dilatation of the intra- and extrahepatic ducts above a stricture of the lower end of the common bile duct, suggesting a carcinoma of the head of the pancreas.

c. Presenting symptoms include:
  - painless jaundice, pruritus, dark urine
  - back pain, possibly with the symptoms of diabetes mellitus.

53.
a. There are sclerotic areas within both femur and tibia.
b. Avascular necrosis.
c. Predisposing conditions include:
  - long-term treatment with steroids
  - sickle cell disease
  - deep sea diving (Caisson disease).

54.
a. A right ventricular shunt has been inserted to relieve hydrocephalus.
b. Shunts may block or become secondarily infected.

55.
a. There is a broad-based pleural opacity in the right midzone with associated bone destruction.
b. Carcinoma of the bronchus or metastatic tumour. The absence of a pleural effusion makes a mesothelioma unlikely.

56.
a. An arteriovenous malformation is evident.
b. Complications include epilepsy and subarachnoid or intracerebral bleeding.

57.
a. This is a left pulmonary angiogram. There is also a Swan–Ganz catheter in the right pulmonary artery.
b. There is absent perfusion to the left upper lobe and filling defects in the left lower lobe branches, indicating pulmonary emboli.
c. Predisposing causes include:
  - immobility
  - surgery, especially pelvic and orthopaedic surgery
  - pregnancy
  - thrombophilic states (e.g. thrombocythaemia, protein C or antithrombin III deficiency, and underlying malignancy)
  - antiphospholipid syndrome (primary or secondary to systemic lupus erythematosus).

58.
a. Both kidneys are hydronephrotic with markedly distended pelvicalyceal systems.
b. Presenting symptoms may include:
  - oliguria or even anuria (the latter suggests either complete bilateral ureteric obstruction or bilateral renal artery occlusion)—note that a partial obstruction may cause polyuria secondary to defective tubular concentration of urine
  - symptoms of uraemia if renal failure is advanced, such as anorexia, nausea, vomiting, hiccoughs or pruritus.
c. Possible causes include:
  - bilateral ureteric obstruction, e.g. calculi or renal papillary necrosis

- retroperitoneal metastatic tumour, including cervical or colonic carcinoma with ureteric obstruction
- retroperitoneal fibrosis
- bladder neoplasms obstructing both ureteric orifices
- benign prostatic hypertrophy.

59.
a. There is collapse of the left upper lobe which is most likely due to a mucus plug.
b. Treatment consists of endotracheal suction, physiotherapy or bronchoscopic lavage.

60.
a. There is gross dilatation of the right pelviureteric system with a normal calibre proximal ureter, while the left kidney is normal. The diagnosis is pelviureteric junction (PUJ) obstruction.
b. It is thought to be due to a ring of collagenous connective tissue at the PUJ, which results in a functional defect of peristalsis of the collecting system but no actual mechanical obstruction. Occasionally, obstruction may be due to an aberrant renal blood vessel.
c. An open or endoluminal pyeloplasty may be beneficial.

61.
a. There is endosteal scalloping of the fourth metacarpal with some expansion of the bone. There is also punctate calcification within the lesion. This is an enchondroma (benign cartilage tumour).
b. A pathological fracture is a common presenting complaint.
c. Yes—over 50% occur in the hands and wrists.

62.
a. Lower limb venogram.
b. There are extensive confluent filling defects throughout a long segment of the femoral vein, indicating a deep venous thrombosis.
c. Anticoagulation with warfarin for 3 months (initially with intravenous heparin) is indicated for 'above-knee' venous thrombosis. However, if the thrombus is not extensive and confined to veins below the knee, then strapping of the leg with compression stockings may be sufficient.

63.
a. There is borderline cardiomegaly together with a prominent pulmonary outflow tract and pulmonary plethora, indicating a left to right intracardiac shunt.
b. The development of atrial fibrillation suggests an atrial septal defect.
c. Physical signs include a wide, fixed, split-second heart sound and a pulmonary flow murmur.
d. Further investigations indicated are:

- an electrocardiograph (to confirm arrhythmia), which reveals right bundle branch block
- an echocardiogram
- a cardiac catheterisation if surgical correction is contemplated.

64.
a. There is bilateral speckled calcification over the renal outlines, indicating nephrocalcinosis. In view of the normal biochemistry, the most likely diagnosis is medullary sponge kidney.

b. Patients with this condiiton may pass small calculi, which, in this instance, has resulted in right renal colic.

65.
a. There is a pericardial effusion with a pericardial drain in situ. In addition, there is an area of consolidation in the left lower lobe.

b. Possible diagnoses include:
- a primary pneumonic illness, e.g. *Streptococcus pneumoniae* or tuberculosis, with spread of the infection to the adjacent pericardial space (purulent pericardial fluid)
- a primary bronchial neoplasm, with consolidation secondary to bronchial obstruction and metastatic spread to the pericardium (blood-stained pericardial fluid).

c. A pericardial drain has been inserted. Microbiological culture and cytological examination of the pericardial fluid are essential.

66.
a. Absent perfusion to the right lung.
b. Pulmonary embolus.
c. She may have presented with chest pain, dizziness (hypotension), haemoptysis, breathlessness, etc.
d. Physical signs include:
- peripheral or central cyanosis
- hypotension, low volume pulse and tachycardia (sinus tachycardia or atrial dysrhythmias)
- elevated jugular venous pressure
- pleural rub
- evidence of a deep venous thrombosis.

67.
a. The gallbladder is full of calculi and there is a filling defect (just above the endoscope) in the dilated common bile duct, suggestive of a stone, together with partial filling of the pancreatic duct.

b. A surgical clip is evident in (B) with no filling of the gall-bladder, indicating that this patient has undergone a laparoscopic cholecystectomy. The marked dilatation of the common hepatic and common bile duct was thought to be secondary to a further stone but no calculus was found.

68.
a. There are numerous ring shadows throughout the right lung.
b. (B) is a bronchogram which elegantly demonstrates numerous cystic areas. This is marked right cystic bronchiectasis. CT scanning has now largely replaced this more invasive technique.
c. Treatment includes the following:
- physiotherapy with daily postural drainage
- antibiotic therapy of intercurrent infections
- therapy with bronchodilators, if there is concurrent airways obstruction
- surgical resection may be possible for localised disease.

69.
a. There is a large aneurysm arising from the terminal right carotid artery.
b. Associated conditions include:
- coarctation of the aorta
- adult polycystic kidney disease
- Ehlers–Danlos syndrome.
c. Surgical clipping.

70.
a. The kidney has been replaced by numerous cysts.
b. Adult polycystic kidney disease (APKD).
c. Treatment consists of meticulous control of hypertension, and renal dialysis/transplantation if renal failure supervenes.

71.
a. There is an opacity behind the cardiac shadow which rises above the left heart border. On the lateral X-ray this is seen to be a tortuous aneurysmal descending aorta. Atheromatous disease is the most likely underlying cause.

72.
a. There is an isodense subdural collection on the right, with midline shift to the left. The grey–white matter interface on the right shows the position of the right parietal cortex. The collection is approximately 2–3 weeks old.
b. The collection could be surgically drained, but in this case it was treated conservatively. Follow-up scans showed slow spontaneous resolution.

73.
a. There is an intertrochanteric fracture of the left femur with separation of the lesser trochanter.
b. The patient will have shortening and external rotation of the left leg, together with marked pain on movement of the left hip.
c. Surgical fixation when the patient is medically fit.

74.
a. There are electrocardiograph electrodes and an oxygen mask evident. In addition, there is cardiomegaly, bilateral pulmonary oedema with fluid in the right horizontal fissure, and marked upper lobe blood diversion.
b. Pulmonary oedema, which is most commonly secondary to acute left ventricular failure.
Treatment includes:
- oxygen
- intravenous opiates, e.g. diamorphine with an anti-emetic
- intravenous boluses of diuretics such as frusemide
- intravenous infusions of nitrates, such as glyceryl trinitrate, to offload the left ventricle if the systolic blood pressure is adequate.
c. Cardiac causes of pulmonary oedema include:
- acute myocardial infarction
- arrhythmias
- severe valvular disease, e.g. aortic stenosis, mitral stenosis or aortic incompetence
- acute myocarditis.

75.
a. The C3/4 disc has been excised and a bone graft inserted. The graft material has become displaced and is indenting the pharynx, as can be seen on the barium swallow image.
b. The patient's symptoms were not sufficiently troublesome to warrant further surgical intervention.

76.
a. The bones are normal but there is very marked vascular calcification.
b. This is most likely to be the result of long-standing insulin-dependent diabetes mellitus, but prolonged renal failure with poor calcium/phosphate control (hence causing the solubility product to be exceeded) can also result in metastatic calcification.

77.
a. There is asymmetrical osteopaenia with a severe compression fracture of an upper thoracic vertebra. Also, there are wedge deformities of varying severity of multiple vertebral bodies.
b. Osteoporosis can produce this type of radiological appearance, but the combination of hypercalcaemia, renal dysfunction, osteopaenia and a compression fracture strongly suggests myeloma.
c. Further investigations include:
- immunoglobulins and serum electrophoresis
- examination for Bence–Jones proteinuria.
d. Treatment includes the following:
- cautious intravenous fluid, if dehydrated, together with

steroids or diphosphonates, which are helpful for hypercalcaemia
- radiotherapy may be used for localised bone disease
- various effective chemotherapy regimens are available, e.g. VAD (vincristine, adriamycin and dexamethasone)
- symptomatic treatment, e.g. analgesia and blood transfusions
- because many patients relapse, high-dose ablative chemotherapy followed by a peripheral blood stem cell transplant may be performed in young patients.

78.
a. There is a filling defect which represents a sessile colonic polyp.
b. The patient should undergo a colonoscopy and polypectomy.

79.
a. The plain scan demonstrates multiple nodules within the brain and posterior fossa, with significant oedema, most marked in the frontal lobes. They enhance significantly in a ring-like pattern after i.v. contrast is administered.
b. These lesions were secondary deposits from a neglected breast primary lesion. Similar appearances can be caused by infective abscesses, but patients are usually more toxic and unwell. In immunocompromised patients, toxoplasma should be excluded.

80.
a. There is a calcaneal spur.
b. Treatment includes:
- local steroid injection
- appropriate footwear
- surgery is occasionally indicated.

81.
a. There is a right-sided hydropneumothorax, i.e. air and fluid in the right pleural cavity.
b. The radiological differential diagnosis consists of:
- rupture of a cavitating pulmonary lesion, e.g. carcinoma or abscess into the pleural space
- trauma with right rib fracture(s) and a secondary haemopneumothorax
- a pneumothorax complicating an aspiration of a pleural effusion or a pleural biopsy.
c. Further investigations include the following:
- insertion of an apical and basal chest drain
- the pleural fluid (transudate, exudate, blood or pus) should be sent off for glucose and protein estimations, microbiological culture (including tuberculosis) and cytological examination for malignant cells
- the chest X-ray must be repeated after drainage of the fluid

to determine if there is an underlying pulmonary lesion; a bronchoscopy or CT scan may be indicated.

82.
a. There is a homogenous triangular opacity within the cardiac shadow, which represents the collapsed left lower lobe. Note that the left hilum is displaced downwards and is therefore indistinct, and there is loss of the medial end of the left diaphragm.

b. Physical signs include the following:
- dullness to percussion at the left base posteriorly
- bronchial breathing will be present if there is any consolidation within the left lower lobe.

c. Causes include mucus plugging, which will usually resolve with physiotherapy. Aspiration of a tooth etc. during anaesthesia, though unlikely, should be considered.

83.
a. There is a large retro-orbital mass with a resultant proptosis of the right eye.

b. Causes include:
- primary retro-orbital tumour such as an optic nerve glioma
- metastatic deposit.

84.
a. There is marked resorption of the terminal phalangeal tuft together with subperiosteal resorption of the phalanges which is maximal on the radial aspect. There is a 'rugger jersey' appearance of the lumbar vertebrae.

b. Advanced renal osteodystrophy secondary to severe tertiary hyperparathyroidism.

c. This patient requires a parathyroidectomy followed by treatment with calcitriol.

85.
a. There is a large area of increased radiolucency affecting the left upper and midzone, which is a large emphysematous bulla. Note the compression of the adjacent lung parenchyma. Right-sided bullae are also present.

b. Physical signs over the bulla include an increased percussion note and reduced breath sounds.

c. Surgery (bullectomy) may be of benefit in selected cases.

86.
a. The early scan shows a well perfused renal transplant overlying the left common iliac artery. The later scan, however, demonstrates a 'photon-deficient' region, i.e. a hole which corresponds to the renal transplant. The transplant has infarcted.

b. There are two possible causes:
- renal artery thrombosis, e.g. secondary to an intimal flap
- renal vein thrombosis.

c. The patient requires a transplant nephrectomy, discontinuation of immunosuppression, and will return to maintenance dialysis.

87.
a. This is a per-operative cholangiogram performed in a patient who is undergoing an open cholecystectomy. Contrast is injected via the cannulated cystic duct, and the free flow of contrast into the duodenum with no filling defects, as in this case, indicates that there are no residual stones within the common bile duct. It is imperative to ensure that the entire length of the common bile duct is adequately visualised.

88.
a. There is marked dilatation of the intrahepatic ducts.
b. Possible causes include:
   - intrinsic obstruction (cholangiocarcinoma, stones)
   - extrinsic obstruction (carcinoma of the head of the pancreas, lymphadenopathy at the porta hepatis).
c. Investigations required include routine blood tests, with blood cultures. The patient should undergo endoscopic retrograde cholangiopancreatography (ERCP) and should be treated with systemic antibiotics and kept well hydrated.

89.
a. There is a double-J stent in situ which extends from the right renal pelvis to the bladder, together with a right nephrostomy tube.
b. This patient has been treated for an acutely obstructed right kidney, initially by insertion of a nephrostomy and subsequently a double-J stent. The history suggests acute renal colic secondary to either a calculus or renal papillary necrosis (which has an increased incidence in diabetic patients). The double-J stent will be removed cystoscopically in a few months' time.

90.
a. There are marked irregularities of both sacroiliac joints with periarticular sclerosis indicating a bilateral symmetrical sacroiliitis.
b. Causes include:
   - ankylosing spondylitis
   - psoriatic arthropathy
   - inflammatory bowel disease, e.g. ulcerative colitis or Crohn's disease.

   Causes of an asymmetrical sacroiliitis include rheumatoid arthritis, osteoarthritis or Reiter's syndrome (a triad of urethritis, conjunctivitis and seronegative arthritis). A unilateral sacroiliitis suggests a possible septic arthritis.

91.
a. There are bilateral renal calculi. In addition, there is a continuous ambulatory peritoneal dialysis catheter (also

called a Tenchkoff catheter) in situ, indicating that the patient has end stage renal failure.

b. The patient may have had primary hyperparathyroidism, complicated by renal calculi and renal failure. Alternatively, the patient may have been an idiopathic stone former and may have developed hyperparathyroidism as a complication of long-standing renal failure.

92.
a. There is a peripheral wedge-shaped opacity in the right midzone.

b. Pulmonary infarct secondary to a pulmonary embolus with early cavitation evident.

c. Other useful investigations include arterial blood gases together with an electrocardiograph. A ventilation–perfusion scan is confirmatory.

93.
a. There are multiple hypoechoic areas within the liver parenchyma.

b. Possible causes include:
- metastases from a primary colonic neoplasm (ulcerative colitis predisposes the individual to adenocarcinoma)
- pyogenic abscesses.

c. Further investigations include:
- fine needle aspiration or biopsy of the hepatic lesions under ultrasound guidance (ensure normal clotting and platelets)
- barium enema or colonoscopy.

94.
a. There is a solid mixed echotexture cortical mass within the renal parenchyma.

b. Hypernephroma.

c. Ectopic production of the hormone erythropoeitin by the tumour.

d. A staging abdominal CT scan to look for involvement of the renal vein and lymph nodes, as well as a chest X-ray. The mainstay of treatment remains surgical.

95.
a. There is marked asymmetry in the excretion of the radioisotope between the right and left kidneys (27 and 73%, respectively), and the right kidney appears smaller.

b. Causes of a smaller, poorly functioning right kidney include:
- congenitally dysplastic kidney
- long-standing ischaemia, secondary to either fibromuscular hyperplasia or atheromatous disease
- intrinsic renal disease such as chronic pyelonephritis
- long-standing unilateral obstruction.

96.
a. There is a peripherally enhancing low attenuation lesion in the left frontal lobe.
b. A cerebral abscess secondary to infective endocarditis.
c. The patient requires:
- treatment with anticonvulsants to try and prevent further fits
- possible neurosurgical referral for formal drainage
- continuation of treatment with systemic antibiotics according to the results of microbiological cultures.

97.
a. The left kidney is of normal size, shape and position. No renal structure is identified in the right upper quadrant, although a distal ureter can be discerned. Close scrutiny reveals contrast-filled calyces over the right side of the sacrum, indicating a right pelvic kidney.
b. No.
c. This patient has significant renal disease which requires further investigations, including:
- autoantibody screen and complement levels (for systemic lupus erythematosus)
- immunoglobulins and Bence–Jones' protein (for myeloma)
- anti-neutrophil cell antibody assay and antiglomerular basement membrane antibody levels (for various vasculitides and anti-GBM disease, respectively)
- percutaneous left renal biopsy.

98.
a. There is a large cavity with an air/fluid level within the superior portion of the right lobe of the liver with several small satellite lesions. The appearance is typical of multiple liver abscesses.
b. Underlying causes include:
- intra-abdominal sepsis (e.g. diverticulitis or appendicitis) with a secondary portal pyaemia
- cholangitis, i.e. sepsis within the (usually obstructed) biliary tree (e.g. gallstones, tumour), but can also result from interventional procedures.
c. This patient requires:
- intravenous broad-spectrum antibiotics
- percutaneous drainage of the abscess cavities with microbiological culture of the material obtained
- removal or other treatment, e.g. stenting of any obstructive lesions when the patient is medically fit.

99.
a. There is a linear soft tissue opacity partly obscuring the right heart border with obliteration of the cardiophrenic angle and a small right hilum, indicating collapse of the right lower lobe.

    b. The patient has probably aspirated a small piece of food
       which has obstructed the right lower lobe bronchus; he
       therefore merits a therapeutic bronchoscopy.

100.
    a. There is a matched defect approximating to the left lower
       lobe.
    b. Causes include:
- pneumonia
- collapse and consolidation secondary to bronchial obstruction.

101.
    a. There are multiple small calcific densities throughout both
       lung fields which are otherwise normal.
    b. Chickenpox pneumonia (varicella zoster) in adulthood.
    c. No.

102.
    a. There are multiple, small, well-defined areas of high signal
       throughout the deep white matter of both cerebral
       hemispheres. Appearances are typical of demyelination
       secondary to multiple sclerosis.
    b. The loss of visual acuity is secondary to either of the
       following:
- an optic neuritis, when the optic disc swelling can be distinguished from papilloedema by the presence of significant visual loss
- a retrobulbar neuritis, where the optic disc may appear normal in the acute instance but will became pale later as a result of optic atrophy. A relative afferent pupillary defect is present and persistent.

103.
    a. There is an irregular liver with splenomegaly and
       considerable ascites.
    b. Cirrhosis.
    c. Causes include:
- idiopathic (the majority)
- ethanolic
- hepatitis B or C infection
- rarer causes such as haemochromatosis, Wilson's disease and alpha-1-antitrypsin deficiency.

    d. Useful investigations include:
- blood tests, including liver function tests, albumin, clotting, ferritin, caeruloplasmin and alpha-1-antitrypsin levels
- hepatitis serology
- ascitic tap (typically a transudate)
- liver biopsy (including staining for iron) after treatment with diuretics to reduce ascites.

104.
a. There is extensive bilateral apical pleural thickening and fibrosis, with subsequent loss of lung volume and bilateral elevation of the hila.
b. Previous pulmonary tuberculosis with no evidence of active disease.

105.
a. The plain X-ray is unremarkable, although the bones are mildy osteopaenic. The isotope bone scan, however, reveals marked uptake over the whole right femoral shaft.
b. Late infection of the prosthesis.

106.
a. (A) shows that the infected hip prosthesis has been removed and gentamicin-impregnated beads have been placed in the hip joint and along the femoral shaft. These beads produce very high local concentrations of gentamicin without the risks of systemic toxicity. (B) shows a definitive surgical fixation after the infection has been eradicated.

107.
a. The striking abnormality is consolidation of the left lower lobe with an adjacent pleural effusion. The diagnosis is left lower lobe pneumonia with a sympathetic effusion. If the patient had a persistent fever despite antibiotic treatment, then an empyema should be considered and the pleural fluid aspirated and sent for culture.
b. Dullness at the left base with bronchial breathing above the effusion.
c. Further investigations include:
  - blood and sputum cultures
  - oxygen saturation or blood gases if carbon dioxide retention is suspected
  - routine haematology and biochemical tests (pneumonias can result in renal failure)
  - consider bronchoscopy if infection does not resolve or if it recurs quickly despite adequate treatment to exclude bronchial obstruction.

108.
a. A left chest drain has been inserted for a pneumothorax and there is gross surgical emphysema with air outlining muscle and fascial planes in the soft tissues. Occasionally, chest drains become malpositioned and allow air to pass from the pleural cavity into the soft tissues. A new chest drain is required. The condition is not dangerous and the air will slowly resorb.
b. The patient may look alarmingly swollen and there will be palpable crepitus over the torso and upper limbs.

109.
a. There is free fluid in the right subhepatic space.
b. The commonest cause is bleeding (splenic or hepatic rupture, mesenteric injury, etc.). An intraperitoneal rupture of the

bladder was found at laparotomy. A seatbelt compressing a distended bladder can result in rupture, either intraperitoneal (surgical repair required) or extraperitoneal (catheter drainage often adequate).

110.
a. The bones have become markedly sclerotic, which suggests widespread bony metastases from a prostatic carcinoma.
b. Further investigations include:
- serum prostate specific antigen (PSA) which may be used to follow response to treatment
- prostatic biopsy to confirm the diagnosis
- routine haematology and biochemistry, e.g. renal failure may result from obstruction to the renal tract at the prostatic or retroperitoneal level.
c. Treatment options include:
- transurethral resection of the prostate if obstruction is present
- bilateral orchidectomy
- attempts at hormonal manipulation with anti-androgens, e.g. stilboestrol, cyproterone acetate
- local radiotherapy for symptomatic localised metastatic disease.

111.
a. There is marked calcification of the right kidney. The history suggests renal tuberculosis with an autonephrectomy.
b. Investigations include:
- three early morning urines for TB culture
- chest X-ray to exclude concomitant pulmonary TB
- Heaf test.

112.
a. There has been a previous left thoracoplasty, as evidenced by the destruction of the left upper ribs. In addition, there has been a left pneumonectomy, as evidenced by an opaque left hemithorax with metallic surgical sutures over the proximal left main bronchus.
b. The thoracoplasty was performed for tuberculosis, while the pneumonectomy could have been performed for ongoing tuberculosis, a bronchial carcinoma or a so-called 'scar carcinoma', which may have arisen in the scar from the previous surgery.

113.
a. Endoscopic retrograde cholangiopancreatography (ERCP).
b. There is a dilated common bile duct with a tight hilar stricture. There is gross dilatation of the hepatic ducts above the stricture.
c. The differential diagnosis includes extrinsic compression

secondary to lymphadenopathy at the porta hepatis, and intrinsic obstruction secondary to cholangiocarcinoma.
d. Stenting of the stricture may provide relief of jaundice and pruritus.

114.
a. There is bilateral hilar enlargement secondary to lymphadenopathy. Pulmonary hypertension is unlikely in view of the normal cardiac silhouette and pulmonary vascular markings.
b. The differential diagnosis includes sarcoidosis and lymphoma.
c. Pulmonary function tests would be normal as there is no involvement of the lung parenchyma.
d. Further investigations include:
   - Sarcoidosis—serum calcium, serum angiotensin-converting enzyme (SACE), bronchoscopy with bronchial or transbronchial biopsy; consider Kveim test and tuberculin test
   - lymphoma—lymph node biopsy, staging imaging of thorax, abdomen and pelvis (usually a combination of CT and ultrasound).

115.
a. There is compression of the cervical spinal cord, which in this case is secondary to cervical spondylosis.
b. Physical signs may include:
   - spastic quadraparesis (note that the tone is flaccid initially in acute cord compression prior to the development of spasticity)
   - a sensory level
   - retention of urine and loss of anal tone secondary to loss of sphincter control.
c. Neurosurgical decompression is the only treatment but has a high morbidity and mortality in such patients.

116.
a. Abnormalities include the following:
   - severe osteoarthritic changes affecting the lumbar vertebrae (florid osteophyte formation) as well as the right hip; there has also been a previous hemiarthroplasty
   - a calcified mass is seen in the pelvis which represents a calcified fibroid
   - a right femoral dialysis catheter is in situ.
b. No.

117.
a. There is widespread mottled pulmonary shadowing, more marked on the right, with loss of lung volume.
b. The association with hypercalcaemia makes sarcoidosis the most likely diagnosis.

   c. Other organs which may be involved in sarcoidosis include:
   - bones (arthralgia, dactylitis)
   - skin (lupus pernio, erythema nodosum)
   - kidney (interstitial granulomatous nephritis, renal calculi, hypercalcaemic nephropathy)
   - central nervous system (cranial/peripheral nerve palsies, diabetes insipidus secondary to pituitary involvement)
   - eyes (iritis, lacrimal gland involvement).
   d. Active ocular, renal or pulmonary disease requires treatment with prednisolone. Other drugs, including hydroxychloroquine, methotrexate and azathioprine, have also been used.

118.
   a. The head of the pancreas is significantly enlarged, of low attenuation and oedematous, with dilatation of the pancreatic duct in the tail of the pancreas. There is adjacent gastric and duodenal compression.
   b. Acute pancreatitis. Predisposing causes include:
   - ethanol
   - gallstones
   - hypercalcaemia
   - viral infections, e.g. Coxsackie virus
   - trauma.
   c. Treatment includes:
   - fluid, electrolyte and nutritional support (patients may require total parenteral nutrition)
   - close radiological follow-up for potential complications including a pancreatic pseudocyst or abscess.

119.
   a. There is severe dilatation (greater than 5 cm) of the descending colon, which is gas-filled, but there is no evidence of perforation. This is toxic megacolon.
   b. Treatment consists of the following:
   - high-dose intravenous steroids
   - intravenous fluids
   - daily abdominal X-rays and abdominal girth measurements
   - a colectomy is indicated if the patient is very unwell or does not settle within 48 hours.

120.
   a. There is severe generalised osteopaenia with a moderate kyphosis and evidence of wedging of vertebral bodies of varying severity.
   b. Osteoporosis.
   c. Predisposing causes include:
   - increasing age
   - treatment with corticosteroids
   - prolonged immobilisation

- early menopause
- thyrotoxicosis.

121.

a. There is complete opacification of the left hemithorax with elevation of the left hemidiaphragm (note the elevated position of the gastric air bubble), indicating complete left lung collapse. There is also tracheal displacement and mediastinal shift to the left, left rib 'crowding' and compensatory over-expansion of the otherwise normal right lung.

b. Possible causes include:
   - intrinsic bronchial obstruction (tumour, foreign object, sputum plug)
   - extrinsic bronchial obstruction (tumour, lymphadenopathy).

   Note that the absence of metallic surgical sutures excludes a left pnemonectomy from the differential diagnosis.

c. Further investigations include:
   - bronchoscopy with biopsy and cytology
   - radiological staging CT scan of thorax
   - assessment of the liver and adrenal glands (CT or ultrasound)
   - full blood count, urea, electrolytes and calcium.

122.

a. There is a large amount of free gas under both diaphragms.

b. The most likely diagnoses in a woman of this age are:
   - perforated peptic ulcer
   - perforation of other abdominal viscera such as colon.

   Note that this appearance may occur after a laparoscopy, laparotomy or penetrating injury.

c. The following are indicated:
   - urea and electrolytes, full blood count and cross match
   - venous access and intravenous fluids
   - antibiotics and H_2 antagonists
   - laparotomy and appropriate surgical procedures.

123.

a. There are large bilateral polycystic kidneys. Adult polycystic kidney disease is autosomal dominant with nearly 100% penetrance, and recently a gene has been identified on chromosome 16.

b. Intracranial berry aneurysms.

c. Complications include:
   - renal failure
   - hypertension
   - haematuria and bleeding into a cyst
   - subarachnoid haemorrhage
   - increased incidence of renal tumours.

124.
  a. There is a very large shadow behind the cardiac silhouette which contains an air–fluid level and is typical of a large sliding hiatus hernia.

125.
  a. The right kidney is small and there is blunting of the calyces, indicating chronic pyelonephritis.

  b. Management consists of monitoring blood pressure and renal function together with the early detection of urinary tract infections. If infections are frequent, long-term prophylactic antibiotics may be required.

126.
  a. There are osteoarthritic changes with loss of joint space and sclerosis particularly affecting the lateral compartment. In addition, there are some calcific opacities lying posteriorly within the joint space.

  b. Intra-articular loose bodies.

  c. The patient may complain of 'locking' or 'giving way' of the knee.

  d. Arthroscopy and removal of the loose bodies.

127.
  a. The pelvicalyceal systems of both kidneys are distorted, suggesting a diagnosis of adult polycystic kidney disease. Ultrasound examination would confirm the presence of bilateral, multiple cysts.

  b. Modes of presentation include:
- macroscopic haematuria
- urinary tract infection
- pain secondary to bleeding into a cyst or 'clot colic'
- hypertension
- via screening if a relative has the condition
- renal failure.

  c. Management consists of monitoring renal function and hypertension which, if present, should be meticulously controlled.

128.
  a. There is loss of the normal glenoid–humeral alignment, the parallel joint lines being lost. The humeral head has a 'light bulb' shape, suggesting a posterior dislocation (4% of shoulder dislocations). The axial projection confirms the posterior displacement of the humeral head.

  b. The dislocation requires closed reduction, with repeat X-rays to confirm satisfactory reduction.

129.
  a. This patient has an endotracheal tube in situ and is therefore ventilated in the intensive care department. There is a bilateral 'ground glass' appearance throughout the lung fields but predominantly affecting the midzones. There is no upper lobe blood diversion, cardiomegaly or Kerley B lines evident.

    b. These features suggest a diagnosis of adult repiratory distress syndrome (ARDS) rather than left ventricular failure or salt and water overload, e.g. secondary to renal failure.

    c. Causes of ARDS include:
- severe sepsis
- aspiration of gastric contents
- severe bacterial or viral pneumonia
- pancreatitis
- massive bleeding or massive transfusion
- major trauma or surgery
- oxygen toxicity.

130.
    a. Yes—there is no significant pulmonary pathology since the opacities are due to calcified costal cartilages.

    b. Chilaiditi's syndrome. There is colonic interposition between the right lobe of the liver and the hemidiaphragm (note that there are colonic haustrations present), which gives the impression of free peritoneal gas.

    c. No further investigations are required.

131.
    a. The left kidney is not identified either because it is completely obstructed or because the patient has had a previous left nephrectomy. The pelvicalyceal system of the right kidney is significantly dilated and the right ureter can be traced to just below the sacroiliac joint where a radio-opaque calculus is evident. In addition, a large staghorn calculus can be discerned within the right kidney.

    b. The following are indicated:
- a midstream urine specimen to exclude active infection
- urea and electrolytes (since obstruction to a single functioning kidney will result in renal failure)
- urgent relief of the obstruction by endoscopic removal of the stone or by the insertion of a nephrostomy.

132.
    a. There is consolidation of the right upper lobe with an air bronchogram, and the most likely diagnosis is a primary infective pneumonic illness.

133.
    a. There is a single thin-walled cavity containing an air–fluid level in the right upper zone which is typical of a lung abscess.

    b. Predisposing conditions include:
- epilepsy and alcoholism (both of which predispose to aspiration of gastric contents and foreign bodies)
- bronchial obstruction with secondary infection
- certain types of pneumonia (e.g. staphylococcal and *Klebsiella*) which are particularly prone to cavitation.

134.
a. There are areas of increased activity throughout the axial skeleton, suggesting multiple metastatic deposits.
b. Tumours which commonly metastasise to bone include adenocarcinoma of the prostate, lung, stomach, colon and breast (although not in this case).
c. Useful investigations include:
- serum calcium
- full blood count to exclude an iron deficiency anaemia secondary to gastrointestinal blood loss
- prostate specific antigen
- plain X-rays of the affected skeleton.

135.
a. There is bilateral dilatation of both pelvicalyceal systems (more marked on the right), with dilatation of the proximal left ureter.
b. Bilateral ureteric obstruction in this patient may be due to retroperitoneal tumour, e.g. metastatic carcinoma of the cervix, breast or gastrointestinal tract, or more rarely retroperitoneal fibrosis. Careful enquiry for gynaecological or gastrointestinal symptoms should be made.
c. The following are indicated:
- routine haematology and biochemistry (for renal function), including ESR which may be elevated in retroperitoneal fibrosis
- abdominal ultrasound or, preferentially, an abdominal CT scan in order to make a detailed assessment of the retroperitoneum.

136.
a. There is marked dilatation of the oesophagus, which contains considerable food residue. The distal end of the oesophagus is narrowed.
b. Achalasia of the oesophagus. Patients may complain of:
- halitosis
- regurgitation of undigested food
- aspiration of food debris into the respiratory tract with a secondary pneumonia
- chest pain, which may result from vigorous asynchronous non-peristaltic contractions.
c. Management includes the following:
- dilatation of the oesophageal sphincter
- a cardiomyotomy (Heller's operation) is of value in patients who remain symptomatic following repeated dilatations.
d. Complications include recurrent chest infections and an increased risk of carcinoma of the oesophagus.

137.
a. Dissection of the thoracic aorta.
b. Contrast is evident within the true lumen of the descending

aorta, while the false lumen contains no contrast, giving rise
to the 'tennis ball' sign.
c. Physical signs include the following:
- asymmetrical pulses with different blood pressures in each arm
- arteries arising from the aorta may be partially or completely occluded with resultant regional ischaemia, e.g. cerebrovascular accident if the carotid artery is compromised
- aortic incompetence may develop.
d. Antihypertensive treatment to control hypertension, and referral for surgery if the patient is medically fit.

138.
a. There is left hilar enlargement with filling of the aortopulmonary window.
b. The differential diagnosis includes:
- carcinoma of the bronchus, where the hilar enlargement may be due to the tumour itself or to involvement of the hilar lymph nodes, or both; this is the most likely diagnosis in this particular patient
- lymphoma, although lymphomas are usually bilateral and asymmetrical
- infection, e.g. histoplasmosis, tuberculosis
- sarcoidosis, although unilateral disease is very uncommon.

139.
a. There is an enormous left soft tissue mass arising within the anterior compartment which replaces most of the muscles in the thigh. The subcutaneous tissue is diffusely thickened secondary to oedema. The history and scan suggest a rapidly growing malignant soft tissue tumour.

140.
a. There are bilateral cervical ribs.
b. The cervical rib is pressing on the lower roots of the left brachial plexus (C8 and T1).
c. Cervical ribs may cause:
- Raynaud's phenomenon
- ischaemic arm pain secondary to pressure upon the subclavian artery
- subclavian vein stenosis.
The majority of ribs, however, are incidental findings.

141.
a. A small, calcified abdominal aneurysm is present adjacent to a heterogeneous left-sided mass which extends into the pelvis. A kidney concentrating contrast is seen in the right side of the pelvis.
b. Diagnoses include:

- left psoas haematoma secondary to rupture of an abdominal aortic aneurysm
- right pelvic kidney or a right-sided renal transplant.
c. Adequate resuscitation followed by surgery.

142.
a. There is a large thin-walled lesion within the left upper zone with central cavitation.
b. The most likely diagnosis is a cavitating lung carcinoma (usually squamous cell carcinoma), but it may represent previous pulmonary scarring, e.g. from tuberculosis. Neoplasia should always be considered in the differential diagnosis of all solid or cavitating pulmonary lesions.

143.
a. There are bilateral low attenuation extracerebral collections. The larger left-sided collection exerts a considerable mass effect with compression of the lateral ventricle. The history suggests a long-standing lesion, and the diagnosis is chronic bilateral subdural collections.
b. Predisposing factors include:
- age-related cerebral atrophy
- alcoholism
- epilepsy
- a head injury, which may have been very minor and may not even be remembered.
c. Neurosurgical intervention (craniotomy and evacuation of collection) may lead to complete recovery.

144.
a. The bladder may be seen centrally, while the renal transplant is situated in the left iliac fossa. Gas bubbles can be seen within the renal transplant.
b. Emphysematous pyelonephritis of the transplant kidney, presumably secondary to a urinary tract infection.
c. This patient requires:
- intravenous fluids and insulin
- broad-spectrum systemic antibiotics (after urine and blood cultures)
- transplant nephrectomy, if the patient does not improve with medical therapy.

145.
a. There is a stenosing 'apple core' lesion in the transverse colon which is almost certainly a carcinoma.
b. Carcinoma of the colon may present with a variety of symptoms including:
- alteration of bowel habit
- weight loss

- overt rectal bleeding or iron deficiency as a result of occult bleeding
- metastatic disease.

c. Surgery.

146.

a. There is an oval calcified mass in the lower right abdomen.
b. In view of the history of renal failure, this mass most likely represents a calcified renal transplant which has failed several years previously.

147.

a. There are multiple cavitating lesions in both midzones, with associated ill-defined consolidation.
b. Tuberculosis.
c. Cavitating pulmonary abscesses, e.g. staphylococcal or *Klebsiella* pneumonia, or Wegener's granulomatosis (a rare disorder characterised by pulmonary granulomata which often cavitate and renal failure).
d. Sputum culture for bacteria and mycobacteria, Heaf test, urine dipstick, routine biochemistry and haematology.
e. Triple antituberculous therapy with appropriate monitoring of chest X-ray, weight, albumin and liver function tests (for drug toxicity).

148.

a. There are grossly abnormal loops of small bowel in the right iliac fossa, with deep mucosal ulceration and cobblestoning. The splenic flexure and descending colon are also involved.
b. Extensive Crohn's disease.
c. Complications include:
- subacute intestinal obstruction
- fistulae formation
- perianal disease
- rectal bleeding (less common than in ulcerative colitis)
- weight loss and malabsorption, e.g. vitamin B_{12} deficiency from involvement of the terminal ileum
- arthritis
- skin lesions, including erythema nodosum and pyoderma gangrenosum.

149.

a. There is a complete obstruction at the upper end of the ureter. A renal transplant is effectively a single functioning kidney, and therefore acute renal failure supervenes if obstruction occurs.
b. Causes include:
- blood clot, especially if a renal biopsy has been performed to confirm graft rejection
- ureteric ischaemia and secondary stenosis.

   c. Treatment includes insertion of a nephrostomy/stent or surgical reimplantation of the ureter.

150.
   a. This is an anterior dislocation of the shoulder. The unopposed action of the pectoral muscles pull the humerus inferiorly and medially so that the humeral head lies in the subcoracoid position. The lateral confirms the 'empty glenoid'.

   b. The patient should have a closed reduction under appropriate sedation and analgesia, and the arm should then be immobilised.

151.
   a. There is a markedly elevated right hemidiaphragm, together with pleural thickening and calcification on the right.

   b. Pulmonary tuberculosis.

   c. Right phrenic nerve crush.

152.
   a. There is opacificaion of the left upper zone with multiple circular radiolucent areas of uniform size.

   b. He has had previous left-sided pulmonary tuberculosis which has been treated with plombage with lucite spheres. The spheres (although other material can also be used) are inserted into the apical pleural space to compress diseased tuberculous lung and allow healing to occur in a similar fashion to a thoracoplasty but without the chest wall deformity associated with the latter.

153.
   a. There is an ulcer crater on the lesser curve of the stomach.

   b. Endoscopy and biopsy of the ulcer are indicated to exclude a carcinoma, followed by treatment with H_2 receptor antagonists.

154.
   a. There is mucosal oedema, ulceration and narrowing of the distal transverse colon, splenic flexure and descending colon. The site is typical for ischaemic colitis.

   b. The management is supportive, as in the majority of cases the process will resolve. Surgery is required in the development of full-thickness gangrene of the affected segment.

   c. The affected bowel may heal with stricturing. A repeat barium study after approximately 6 weeks should be considered.

155.
   a. The main abnormality is a marked out-pouching of the artery. Just beyond this aneurysm is a stenosis with a filling defect, indicating thrombus.

   b. A mycotic aneurysm.

   c. Peripheral embolisation.

    d. The affected portion of the artery requires surgical excision and appropriate bypass.

156.
    a. There is an irregular polypoidal lesion, resulting in narrowing of the oesophagus.

    b. Carcinoma of the oesophagus. Tumours are usually squamous cell carcinomas, but adenocarcinomas occur in the lower third where they may arise in a Barret's oesophagus (localised areas of columnar epithelium secondary to reflux oesophagitis). Endoscopy and biopsy allow histological confirmation.

    c. Surgery is limited to those with localised tumour but carries significant morbidity and mortality, while radiotherapy and chemotherapy are of limited use. Treatment is mainly directed at relief of symptoms and includes oesophageal dilatation and stenting in order to relieve dysphagia.

157.
    a. The first metatarsophalangeal joint is grossly abnormal, with marked destruction of bone and with numerous small periarticular bone fragments evident.

    b. Chronic osteomyelitis, which is most common in patients with long-standing diabetes mellitus.

    c. Treatment consists of the following:
- surgical debridement of infected non-viable tissue, which is occasionally combined with the insertion of gentamicin beads, giving very high local concentrations of antibiotic without significant systemic absorption and potential side-effects
- treatment, possibly prolonged, with oral or intravenous antibiotics
- meticulous diabetic control
- consider angiography (with or without angioplasty or surgery) if peripheral vascular disease is present with resultant lower limb ischaemia.

158.
    a. There are numerous calcified lesions throughout the soft tissues which are aligned in the direction of muscle planes.

    b. Cysticercosis, which is contracted by eating badly cooked pork contaminated with the eggs of the tapeworm *Taenia solium*.

    c. CT brain scan to assess the number and position of intracranial lesions.

    d. Treatment includes anticonvulsants and anti-helminthic drugs together with dexamethasone to reduce any cerebral oedema developing around the cysts during the treatment period.

159.
    a. There is a smoothly tapering narrowing of the distal oesophagus which is typical of a peptic stricture. There is also spillage of contrast into the left bronchial tree.

   b. Management consists of:
- endoscopic dilatation
- treatment with H_2 receptor blockers or proton pump inhibitors in order to prevent further reflux oesophagitis.

160.
a. There are loops of dilated small bowel in the lower abdomen, indicating small bowel obstruction. Air in the biliary tree can be discerned.
b. The appearances are of gallstone ileus. The gallstone has perforated from the gallbladder into the duodenum and has subsequently impacted in the distal small bowel. Surgery is required to relieve the obstruction.

161.
a. Contrast has been injected via a direct puncture into the left pelvicalyceal system and demonstrates complete obstruction at the upper ureter.
b. A formal nephrostomy must be inserted in order to relieve the obstruction pending further investigations. Broad-spectrum antibiotics are required pending microbiological culture of the urine, which is mandatory.

162.
a. The patient has had a mitral valve replacement.
b. Physical signs may include a malar flush, atrial fibrillation and a prosthetic first heart sound.
c. Antibiotic prophylaxis must be given prior to invasive procedures, which may result in a transient bacteraemia such as dental work, cystoscopy, colonoscopy, etc.

163.
a. There is aneurysmal dilatation of the visualised segment of the lower abdominal aorta. The iliac arteries are tortuous and the right internal iliac artery is completely occluded.
b. Renovascular disease.
c. The patient may complain of:
- intermittent claudication
- cold peripheries
- impotence
- abdominal pain secondary to mesenteric ischaemia (postprandial angina).

164.
a. There are large bilateral circular opacities in the lower zones.
b. Bilateral mammary implants.

165.
a. There is a well-defined cystic lesion in the head of the pancreas.
b. Carcinoma of the pancreas, which may be confirmed by a CT-guided biopsy.
c. Surgery may be of benefit, depending on the size and location of the tumour.

166.
a. There has been a right hip arthrodesis.
b. As a result of the right hip surgery and the resultant leg shortening, the contralateral hip is more liable to develop degenerative changes. The left hip joint has marked osteoarthritic changes with sclerosis and loss of the joint space.

167.
a. There is deviation of the trachea to the right in the upper mediastinum, with bilateral apical pleural thickening and calcification. There has been a surgical resection of several upper right ribs.
b. Pulmonary tuberculosis.
c. Right-sided thoracoplasty. The rationale behind the operation was to compress an area (usually apical) of cavitating tuberculous lung tissue in order to obliterate the cavities and allow healing to occur.

168.
a. This is a poor inspiratory film with cardiomegaly, but there is clearly a well-defined rounded mass in the superior mediastinum with lateral displacement and compression of the trachea resulting in stridor.
b. Large retrosternal goitre.
c. Lung function tests, T4 and TSH.
d. Surgery.

169.
a. There is significant accumulation of labelled white cells throughout the whole of the large bowel and rectum.
b. Ulcerative colitis affecting the entire colon (pancolitis).

170.
a. There is extensive free peritoneal fluid and a completely disrupted spleen.
b. Resuscitation followed by emergency surgery.

171.
a. There is consolidation of the right lower lobe with an air bronchogram. This lady has an acute lobar pneumonia.
b. Investigations required include blood and sputum cultures, arterial blood gases, atypical serology, full blood count and serum electrolytes, urea and creatinine. Treatment primarily consists of broad-spectrum intravenous antibiotics, oxygen and physiotherapy.

172.
a. In (A) there is huge cardiomegaly which has a globular configuration; this has been reduced considerably in (B).
b. Massive pericardial effusion, which has been drained by ultrasound-guided aspiration (pericardiocentesis).
c. Causes of a pericardial effusion include the following:
   - consequent to an infective pericarditis, e.g. Coxsackie virus or tuberculosis

- Dressler's syndrome (pericarditis following a myocardial infarction)
- connective tissue diseases, e.g. rheumatoid arthritis
- malignant or uraemic pericarditis.

173.
a. Pregnancy must always be considered and excluded.
b. The scan shows a large mass inferior to a normal uterus, with distension of the vagina. This is a case of haematocolpos, where an imperforate hymen leads to the collection of menstrual products.
c. The hymen was incised and 500 ml of blood was drained.

174.
a. There is extensive interstitial basal fibrosis.
b. Fibrosing alveolitis.
c. Causes include:
- cryptogenic fibrosing alveolitis, i.e. idiopathic
- connective tissue disorders, e.g. rheumatoid arthritis, systemic lupus erythematosus, systemic sclerosis, etc.
- extrinsic allergic alveolitis, e.g. farmer's lung, bird fancier's lung.
d. Physical signs include:
- central cyanosis
- finger clubbing
- bilateral, fine, end inspiratory crackles.

175.
a. There is bilateral hyperinflation with formation of bullae and there are flat hemidiaphragms, indicating emphysema.
b. This radiological picture in such a young patient suggests alpha-1-antitrypsin deficiency and also that the patient was a cigarette smoker. Alpha-1-antitrypsin is a glycoprotein which is synthesised in the liver and inhibits proteolytic enzymes (proteases), and therefore individuals with low levels of alpha-1-antitrypsin are prone to protease-mediated damage which occurs particularly in the lungs.
c. Autosomal dominant, with the most severe disease occurring in patients who are homozygotes.
d. Affected individuals can develop cirrhosis of the liver.
e. Treatment includes:
- stopping smoking
- domiciliary oxygen and conventional treatment for chest infections, right heart failure, etc.
- heart–lung transplantation.

176.
a. There is a fracture of the distal radius, producing a 'dinner fork' deformity.
b. Colles' fracture.
c. Predisposing conditions include:

- any condition resulting in weakening of the bones, e.g. osteoporosis
- any condition which may result in falls, e.g. sick sinus syndrome.

177.
a. There is a lobular, intermediate signal, predominantly left-sided paraspinal mass with adjacent bony destruction of vertebral bodies and preservation of the intervening disc. The combination of clinical and radiological findings strongly suggests a cold tuberculous abscess.

178.
a. There is a very large brain stem tumour based upon the pons and extending into the midbrain. Anteriorly, the tumour completely encases the basilar artery which is evident as a dark line running through the tumour. Such tumours are usually regarded as inoperable and may be treated with radiotherapy.

179.
a. There is increased sclerosis in the distal radius. There is also a 'sun-ray' pattern of periosteal reaction. The appearances are typical of an osteogenic sarcoma.
b. The patient should be referred without delay to a specialist bone tumour centre for accurate staging. Inappropriate biopsy may compromise a limb-saving surgical excision.

180.
a. There is a left subclavian dialysis catheter in situ, indicating that he is on dialysis, together with bilateral ground glass alveolar shadowing without signs of fluid overload.
b. This appearance together with the history strongly suggests an opportunistic infection, and urgent microbiological examination of induced sputum or bronchoalveolar lavage fluid is required. Treatment may then be directed at the relevant pathogen, e.g. high-dose co-trimoxazole for *Pneumocystis carinii* pneumonia (with monitoring of sulphamethoxazole levels in view of his renal failure). Patients may need ventilatory support.

181.
a. The entire sacrum is abnormally expanded, with coarse, dense, sclerotic texture to the bone.
b. Paget's disease.
c. The serum alkaline phosphatase is often markedly elevated secondary to the increased bone turnover. The gamma-glutamyl transpeptidase is normal since the elevated alkaline phosphatase is the bone isoenzyme. Calcium and phosphate are also normal.
d. Complications of Paget's disease include:
  - nerve compression, resulting, for example, in deafness
  - pathological fractures through weakened bones

- sarcomatous change and high output cardiac failure, but these are rare.

182.
a. There is a depressed right frontal skull vault fracture, with a small accompanying subdural collection of blood.
b. Neurosurgical transfer for elevation of the fracture fragments and wound toilet comprise the immediate management. Antibiotic therapy and prophylactic anticonvulsants could be instituted prior to transfer.
c. Epilepsy and personality change.

183.
a. There is a single ill-defined hypoechoic lesion within the liver parenchyma.
b. The differential diagnosis includes:
  - pyogenic hepatic abscess—this is most likely in view of the history
  - cavitating primary or secondary tumour.
  The lesion is not typical of a simple cyst and does not have the complicated internal echo pattern of a hydatid cyst.

184.
a. This is a hysterosalpingogram, where contrast is injected through the cervix into the uterus. The uterus is outlined normally and there is filling of the left Fallopian tube with free peritoneal spill. There is no tubal filling on the right.
b. Causes include:
  - pelvic inflammatory disease
  - endometriosis
  - previous tubal surgery, e.g. ectopic pregnancy.

185.
a. There is a filling defect and obstruction to the cranial flow of contrast. CT and MRI scans have superseded myelography as the imaging mode of choice in patients with symptoms suggestive of spinal cord or other central neurological disease.
b. The most likely diagnosis is a tumour of the spinal cord.

186.
a. There is cardiomegaly and upper lobe blood diversion, together with a large circular opacity in the right midzone which does not look dissimilar to a neoplasm. On the lateral X-ray, however, the opacity is seen to consist of encysted fluid within the horizontal fissure. This is the so-called 'vanishing tumour', since it disappears when the cardiac failure is treated.
b. Treatment with standard drugs for cardiac failure is indicated, e.g. diuretics, angiotensin-converting enzyme inhibitors, etc.

Index